"I have always been on the lookout for s: ⬚⬚ ge
lives. This book, and its concept of ele ⬚⬚ ig
invitation to look at our bodies, our he⬚⬚⬚, ⬚⬚⬚ ⬚⬚⬚ world around us as
electric. What I love about this book is the easy to use tools and exercises that empower people to raise their voltage, which translates into
more energy, focus and authentic empowerment." **—Tony Robbins**

"Eileen McKusick is a true pioneer in the field of energy medicine. With
Electric Body, Electric Health, she has written the definitive primer on the
electric nature of the human body, emotions, and life itself. Empowering, easy-to-understand, and at times mind-blowing, this book will
change the way you see yourself and the world."
        —Jack Canfield, coauthor of the #1 *New York Times* bestselling
                Chicken Soup for the Soul series and The Success
                    Principles, and a featured teacher in The Secret

"*Electric Body, Electric Health* is an electrifying read. Indispensable information for everyone who has ever wondered how our body works,
and even what it is made of. . . . Read it, it's for the sake of your electric
health."   **—Ervin Laszlo**, author of *Reconnecting to the Source* and
                        The Immutable Laws of the Akashic Field

"In this remarkable book, Eileen McKusick shares the true nature of our
existence as electrical beings and how simple it can be to transform our
physical, mental, and emotional health. These powerful and effective
methods are simple enough for anyone to follow to improve their health
dramatically. More than ever before, the world needs the information it
contains. I highly recommend you read it and put it to good use to raise
your voltage today." **—Dr. Bradley Nelson**, author of *The Emotion Code*
                            and creator of the Body Code

"In *Electric Body, Electric Health*, Eileen McKusick offers brilliant wisdom that is practical, and life-changing. 'Thinking electrically' is
the missing piece in our understanding of our health and our world.

This enlightening read puts you on the front edge of the bioelectricity revolution—don't miss it!"

—**Marci Shimoff**, #1 *NY Times* bestselling author of *Happy for No Reason* and *Chicken Soup for the Woman's Soul*

"Every now and then you read something that feels so true, you think how is it that science and popular culture doesn't know this? *Electric Body, Electric Health* is one of those books. Like most pioneers in life, Eileen Day McKusick's simple brilliance stems out of necessity, open-mindedness, and a relentless commitment to the groundbreaking truth she was discovering. For anyone who is tired of the maze of supplements or the rigor of meticulous diet, this 'hack,' written in an accessible, personable voice, may just provide more health on every level."

—**Tama Kieves**, *USA Today* featured visionary catalyst and bestselling author of *Thriving Through Uncertainty* and *A Year Without Fear*

"Eileen McKusick is that rare integration of a fearless scientific voyager with the compassionate heart and expertise of an extraordinary healer. In this brilliant book, Eileen weaves together scientific and practical insights on the nature of your Electric Self. In doing so, she urges you to augment your healing capacity, and shine as your brilliant, unencumbered self, in a time where it is so greatly needed. Highly recommended!"

—**Shamini Jain**, Ph.D., Founder & CEO, Consciousness and Healing Initiative, author of *Healing Ourselves*

"Continuing the work of her first book, Eileen furthers the critical task of counteracting the influence of materialism on modern medicine. She takes a major step forward, in the spirit of Walter Russell and Nikola Tesla, by integrating consciousness, aether, plasma, and electricity into a new paradigm that relates equally well to cosmology and biology. She then gives us a map of the body's bioelectric field in order to better understand our own personal health challenges. This book is as useful as it is thought provoking." —**Dr. Andrew Kaufman**

"Ongoing discoveries in diverse branches of the sciences make it clear that Western biomedicine has had a limited understanding of the nature of the human body and what it takes to create and sustain health. In *Electric Body, Electric Health,* Eileen Day McKusick illuminates one of the primary domains missing from the pages of modern medicine: the human biofield and its electric nature. In these pages, she shares with us her own discoveries of the anatomy and functioning of the human biofield and places it front and center in its profound role in maintaining our health and overall well-being. She simultaneously weaves in supportive evidence from biology, physics, and cosmology. As a scientist working in the field of mind/body medicine for many years, I particularly value the sections describing linkages of how properly expressed emotions serve to maintain the health of the biofield and consequently our overall electric health. Eileen is fond of saying to people, "You are amazing!" because she sees the remarkable beings that we are. Start believing it and let your electric nature begin to radiate."

—**Paul J. Mills**, Ph.D., Professor and Chief, Family Medicine and Public Health, and Director of the Center of Excellence for Research and Training in Integrative Health, the University of California at San Diego and Director of Research for the Deepak Chopra Foundation

"An ancient phrase inscribed on the frontispiece of the Temple of Delphi read "Know Thyself." In *Electric Body, Electric Health,* Eileen McKusick helps us all understand, "we are electromagnetic beings bathed in an electrically connected reality." Eileen shares with us how to raise our voltage, through electromagnetic solutions, for better health of our body, mind, and spirit. Everything is energy, and through this beautifully written book, we learn how to bolster our energy, so that we can indeed come closer to the state of awareness, that we 'Know Thyself.'"

—**Dr. Steven A. Ross**, CEO of World Research Foundation

"Eileen McKusick teaches us to 'think electrically' in her stunning new book *Electric Body, Electric Health.* She turns the world of energy healing on its head by proving the point that we are electric beings in an electric

universe before we are biochemical. In it are all the concepts and techniques that you need to learn to raise your voltage enough to live a life of optimal mental, emotional, and physical health. As always, Eileen's work is brilliant, cutting-edge, and eminently practical."   —**Lisa Campion**, author of
The Art of Psychic Reiki and *Energy Healing for Empaths*

"*Electric Body, Electric Health* turns conventional approaches to healing the mind and body upside down and inside out! And it's about time! I got chills reading this as it fills in a most essential piece of the healing puzzle. And it's a smooth read as Eileen McKusick conveys complex principles with understandability, wisdom, and wit. If you're trying everything to feel better and not making the progress you'd like, this book is definitely for you."   —**Kris Ferraro**, author of *Energy Healing* and *Manifesting*

"Eileen's pioneering research ushers in a new paradigm of thought that marries science and spirituality, for the sake of pursuing whole health. Through direct experience, Eileen guides the reader through a revolutionary shift in perspective, that we are fundamentally electromagnetic and vibrational. I would thoroughly recommend this book for anyone seeking tools for personal growth and healing—it is a blue print for reclaiming your power, creative authorship, and electrical sovereignty."

—**Isaac Koren**, cofounder of The Brothers Koren and Your Big Voice

"*Electric Body, Electric Health* by Eileen McKusick reveals a deep yet easy to understand expression of her wisdom and long years of experience in exploring and mapping the biofield of the human system. Eileen gives us easy access to simple truths about our electric body and how to tune it and harmonize it. Her unique perspectives in combination with a fun loving, 'don't take yourself too serious' approach gives new levels of insight to our health and wholeness and teaches us how to take these back in our own hands. I absolutely love her work and highly recommend it to anyone wanting to uplevel their abundance, creativity, potential, well-being, and fulfillment. Eileen is a true master, and reading and practicing her techniques is life-changing."   —**Professor Jeralyn Glass**, musician and Alchemy Crystal
Sound Healing Pioneer

"The concepts and techniques Eileen McKusick describes in her book *Electric Body, Electric Health* have their roots in the ancient techniques of shamanic culture. As a representative of the Sakha (Arctic Siberian) culture, I view this modern description of the electric body as an example of the extraordinary skill of our shamans. The modern Western scientific view often leads to a demystification of the magic within and around us. This pioneering work gives us great opportunity to reawaken our inner healers while connecting to a modern perspective."   —**Zarina Kopyrina**, cofounder of OLOX music project, innovator in the creation of Arctic Beatbox, and pioneer in the development of NEOshamanic healing.

"Eileen Day McKusick's new book empowers the reader with the awareness of their own power and helping them to harness it to achieve a better functioning, happier, higher voltage version of themselves."

—**Rashid A Buttar**, DO, FAAPM, FACAM, FAAPM, Medical Director, Centers for Advanced Medicine

ELECTRIC BODY, ELECTRIC HEALTH

Also by Eileen Day McKusick

Tuning the Human Biofield

ELECTRIC BODY, ELECTRIC HEALTH

Using the Electromagnetism
Within (and Around) You to Recharge,
Rewire, and Raise Your Voltage

EILEEN DAY McKUSICK

ST. MARTIN'S
ESSENTIALS
NEW YORK

First published in the United States by St. Martin's Essentials,
an imprint of St. Martin's Publishing Group

ELECTRIC BODY, ELECTRIC HEALTH. Copyright © 2021 by Eileen Day McKusick. All rights reserved. Printed in the United States of America. For information, address St. Martin's Publishing Group, 120 Broadway, New York, NY 10271.

www.stmartins.com

Designed by Steven Seighman

The Library of Congress Cataloging-in-Publication Data is available upon request.

ISBN 978-1-250-26214-1 (trade paperback)
ISBN 978-1-250-26215-8 (ebook)

Our books may be purchased in bulk for promotional, educational, or business use. Please contact your local bookseller or the Macmillan Corporate and Premium Sales Department at 1-800-221-7945, extension 5442, or by email at MacmillanSpecialMarkets@macmillan.com.

First Edition: 2021

10 9 8 7

CONTENTS

PREFACE: All the Light We Can and Cannot See

On the winter solstice in December of 2009, my son Quinn came to the dinner table and asked my husband and me if we knew that there was a fourth state of matter called *plasma*—the electrically charged gas that makes up as much as 99.99 percent of space, connecting stars, planets, and entire galaxies in vast webs of light. Up until that point, I had learned about only three states of matter: solid, liquid, and gas. How had I missed an entire state of matter? Especially one that, as I would learn, was actually everywhere I looked. That simple question led me down a rabbit hole of discovery, consequently changing the course of my research, work, and entire cosmological worldview.

At that time, I was twenty pounds overweight; broke; deep in debt; suffering with chronic back pain, miserable digestion, acne, an entire colony of plantar warts on my feet, and a stormy marriage; and juggling work, parenting, and being a full-time, first-time college student simultaneously. This theme of struggle on every front had remained entrenched since I first began my journey into health and human potential at age eighteen, and despite decades of reading great piles of self-help books and attending workshops and availing myself of many different forms of healing, I had yet to become fit, abundant, and content. Not even close.

Discovering plasma opened up the door to a whole new world—a world of light and connection, rather than the dark and disconnected, mechanical worldview I had been educated into. It also dovetailed perfectly and synchronistically with the questions I was studying at that time in my master's program and seeking to answer through academic and scientific channels. After spending the previous fifteen years as a sound therapist and independent researcher exploring how the pure coherent tones produced by tuning forks impacted human health and well-being, I had made many inexplicable observations that I was hoping a deep dive into the world of science would shine some light on.

And shine it did! This sudden illumination of the fundamental electrical aspect of our bodies and our electrical connection to the world around us, which I will spell out in this book, revealed the big picture that I had been searching for. It connected the dots of all my previous explorations of sound and vibration, science and spirituality, health and human potential. Once I was able to take it all in, I realized that this recognition of the connected light in all things—from a scientific perspective and not just a spiritual or religious one—was what I had been looking for all along. I had "seen the light" in a way that satisfied both my rational mind and my soul, and my seeking days were over.

Shortly after spending months learning everything I could about plasma (I actually turned it into an independent study for my master's degree), I began to teach the sound therapy method I had developed to my first group of students. Back in 1996, I had introduced a set of "tuning forks for healing" into my then part-time massage therapy practice. Through curiosity and exploration, I somewhat accidentally discovered a unique therapeutic approach, now called Biofield Tuning: a simple, noninvasive, and efficient method that uses tuning forks on and around the body, effectively "tuning" out-of-tune bodies. Through the use of the coherent sound input of the tuning forks, I had stumbled upon an elegant way to release energetic blockages, thereby producing profound and powerful outcomes on the physical, mental, and emotional levels. After almost fifteen years of using this method on clients and watching them grow lighter and brighter and healthier as a result of the work, with my new students, I finally had the opportunity to receive sessions myself.

Almost instantly, my ailments began to heal from receiving "tune-ups."

The plantar warts were among the first to go. My frozen energy started to find its way back into circulation, my own inner voltage began to rise, and I slowly but surely began to solve all the problems I had been confounded by. Now that I had this new awareness, this new force of nature to use as a resource, things started shifting in a powerful way. It was as if my expanding inner light illuminated the world around me, allowing me to perceive solutions and make connections that I had previously been unable to notice.

Those two seemingly disconnected events—discovering the electrical nature of life and beginning to train students in the sound healing method I'd been practicing for so many years—converged to cause a sea change in my life. Through the process of learning a new cosmological story of light and connection, and through receiving tunings from my new students, my perspective on health, life, and the universe as a whole widened to a degree that I never knew possible. I began recognizing other potentialities of thought, feeling, and action that I had previously not even considered, which led to new and effective outcomes rather than the same old circles I had been stuck in.

While I have made use of tuning forks and the practice of Biofield Tuning to get my energetic house in order, I don't want this to be one of those books that is a sales pitch for classes and tools and whatnot (although I do have plenty of those things to supply to you should you desire to make use of them). What I have learned the most from this journey is how to use my own mind—which is to say, my own biofield—more clearly, more efficiently, and more healthfully. Your energy field is a map of your mind, and fundamentally, your mind is the most powerful tool you have. I will provide you with plenty of tips and practices to get your mind in better order, as well as to make your energy stronger, lighter, brighter, and more resilient. In turn, your body will follow.

Essentially, I have unwittingly figured out a hack in the game of life that, when understood and applied, makes it far easier to boost your health, inner and outer wealth, and creative ability. It has two primary components: understanding electricity and working with our emotions. Our emotions and feelings are just electromagnetic waves that naturally pass through our beings like waves in the ocean—unless, that is, we deny, suppress, or repress them, in which case they become frozen and stuck in our bodies and biomagnetic fields and create resistance and static that block the healthy flow of energy. We make our electric bodies stronger and more coherent primarily through effective emotional management (and other simple approaches), and in the pages that follow, I will go in depth into both of these topics.

Today, as I write this on the winter solstice of 2019, I am sitting with my feet in the sand on the beach in Negril, Jamaica, across from my husband of twenty-three years, having weathered many storms together. I have morphed back from my middle-age spread to the fit, trim body I had as a teenager, which I keep not through working out or religiously eating clean but from using sound in a clever way and from mastering the practice of what I call *moderate hedonism* (we will talk about these, too!).

I am out of debt and out of pain, can eat whatever I want and not get fat, do what I love with people I love, and enjoy high levels of energy. I've grown a thriving, global business that has given me the freedom to travel, one of my great loves, and more recently, to turn my focus back to research and music—the things I am really passionate about.

I say all of this not to blow my own horn but to share with you my own journey from scraping coins together to put gas in my $800 Subaru in the mountains of Vermont while my muffin top was hanging out over my thrift-store jeans, to finding the information and illumination I needed to untie the complex knots that I was bound in—the knots that bind us all in some way, and keep us from being liberated to our potential.

The information that I am going to share with you comes from both my own observations from my clinical practice as well as my research into some exciting new fields of science. This information enabled me to "level up" in the game of life, and this book is an invitation for you to do the same: to build an intrinsic awareness of your own light, to focus on raising your voltage and brilliantly shining on the world around you, and to use the light of your own inner illumination to see new solutions to old problems for yourself and for others. We do that by giving ourselves permission to recharge, to follow our "ahhhs," to express our truth, and to have the courage to go with our guts.

While I am a sound therapist and a researcher, I am more fundamentally a teacher. I have my master's degree in integrative education, which sounds rather vague but is actually a very good description of what I do. I teach people how things connect. What I hear from my students all the time is that understanding themselves as electrical beings has helped them to connect the dots between what's going on in their lives and their health on every level. It enhances our awareness of how everything is connected and helps us to identify and target the root causes of our problems. One of my students said it was like "finally peeking behind the veil."

The fundamental truth is that you are the light you are seeking. You are already enlightened, as your biological reality is that you are a being of light, down to your DNA, your cells, and the trillions of biophotons that permeate your entire being. Even your bones, the densest part of your physical being, are piezoelectric crystalline structures that make electricity (light) when they are compressed. And this light that powers you is the same light that powers the sun and the stars, the lightning and the lightning bugs, and the cosmos in its entirety. We are electromagnetic beings bathed in an electrically connected reality.

This is what we will discuss in depth in this book as we shine light on a new understanding of reality that will change your perspective and change your life, just like it has changed my life and many others. Together, we are the way out of these seemingly dark times.

You are vast. You contain multitudes. What has been obstructing that knowing and being is just a story; distorted waves in space that can be tuned back to their underlying harmonious perfection. Beneath the noise in the signal and stories of victimhood and struggle, you are simply one with the unified field, the cosmos itself—you are the universe. And from that perspective, anything is possible.

INTRODUCTION:
Raise Your Voltage

The prevailing paradigm in Western science says that we are chemical, mechanical beings. But a new paradigm is beginning to emerge that suggests that we are fundamentally electromagnetic and vibrational. It suggests that we—and the cosmos that is our home—are made up of light and sound and waveforms across an unimaginably vast array of frequencies.

Like fish in water, we are swimming at all times in a vast ocean of energy. Look around you: Everything is energy! Everything you see is part of the electromagnetic spectrum. Not only light bulbs and computers and iPhones but planets, animals, stars, and entire galaxies—it's all electrical. The page you're reading, the chair you're sitting in, the ground beneath your feet, the planet you live on, the sun that heats that planet are ultimately just electromagnetic energy vibrating at different frequencies—in other words, electricity. It's all energy, frequency, and vibration. Every single thing in our observable universe is in constant motion on an atomic or subatomic level—even things like rocks that appear motionless. As the great physicist Richard Feynman says, "Everything jiggles," or as I like to put it, "Everything jitterbugs," thanks to the exchange of positive and negative forces that gives rise to this dance of energy.

There's no such thing as a "noun" when we get right down to it, because everything is actually a *process*. (Interestingly, the Hopi language doesn't contain any nouns, and it better reflects the essential fluidity of the world around us.) When vibrations come together, they start to sync up and resonate at the same frequency in a kind of spontaneous self-organization—which is described in physics as *sympathetic resonance*. This resonance may also form the basis of what we call *consciousness*, or intelligence, which science is increasingly revealing to be a fundamental property of energy and, therefore, all matter.

Despite the advances of quantum physics, bioelectricity, and other growing branches of science, it is squarely at the question of *energy* that we hit the dividing line between science and spirituality. There is no agreed-upon, standard definition of the energy referred to in energy medicine—specifically so-called subtle energy, the stuff that makes up our human energy field and, perhaps, in varying densities, all of life and the universe. Without a clear definition, and lacking tools sensitive enough to reliably measure subtle energy, it has been relegated to the domain of spirituality.

This divide between science and spirituality has troubled me since I began my journey into health and well-being in my teenage years. I like to think of myself as a *bothist,* and I practice what I call *bothism:* I choose to see things in *both/and* rather than *either/or* terms, shades of gray over black and white. When it comes to matters of science and spirit, we divide up into our ideological camps, a lot of words get thrown around, and a lot of confusion gets created. But really, what the heck are we all talking about? And is it possible that we're actually just using different words to describe the same things? Could it be that what religion calls *spirit* and *soul* and science calls *electricity* are really one and the same? In this book, we are going to explore the idea that we are living in an electromagnetically connected universe and that, ultimately, it's all one light, one electricity, one Source energy, one universal magnetic field, spinning itself into all the light we can and cannot see.

For many years in my sound therapy practice, I was treating people's physical and mental problems by working in their energy fields, also known as the *biofield*. My skeptical, ever-curious mind quickly led me to a deep and long-running investigation of what the heck I was actually working with. What was clear was that when we refer to this invisible substance called *energy* in the context of energy medicine, we are speaking of *electromagnetic energy* as opposed to other kinds of energy (kinetic, thermal, chemical, and so on). So what is electromagnetism? Simply put, it's the movement of charged electric particles and the magnetic fields that are generated from that electric charge. In other words, it's the spectrum of visible and invisible light (or put another way, sound—but we'll get back to that).

But when I started to dig deeper into my understanding of electricity, I came across an interesting problem. There was a lot of confusing and conflicting information. My friend Dr. Dean Radin, a pioneering parapsychologist with the Institute of Noetic Sciences, said to me, "Eileen, no one really understands electricity—and let me know if you find someone who actually does!" If you ask most people what electricity is, they will cite the standard definition that we all learned in school: electricity is the flow of electrons along a wire. According to some perspectives, electrons don't exist at all! Another perspective points out that these alleged electrons actually don't even move through a wire in a closed, alternating current circuit. They stay in one place and jiggle back and forth while the electric force moves bidirectionally *in a field around the wire*. I have come to understand that this simple omission of the *field* aspect of electric current is a big part of the problem with understanding it, as well as understanding the field of energy that moves around our own bodies.

But there are other problems as well. For one thing, electricity isn't just confined to flowing along the wires that power our phones and computers and other modern technologies. It is actually everywhere around us and present in many things that we often don't realize, such as the air, the sun, the solar wind, lightning, the ground under our feet, the bacteria in our guts, and actually our entire bodies, as we will see.

Another omission in our understanding of electricity comes from the idea that electromagnetic waves do not require a medium to propagate through. Light, we are told, travels through the empty vacuum of space. But this was not always believed to be the case. Early explorers of electricity, including Nikola Tesla, understood electricity, or light, as the movement of energy through the *aether*—the all-pervasive "luminiferous ocean of clear light" that these waves traveled through. I have come to see that it is the removal of this unified field of pure potential (which we will explore in much greater depth) that seems to be a big source of the confusion about the nature of electricity and its omnipresence in our natural environment.

Imagine trying to study waves in the ocean without acknowledging the water that the waves are moving through! In our exploration of electricity, we are going to bring two new states of matter into the equation—plasma and aether—which will help give us a better understanding of the nature of our bodies, minds, and the world around us and ultimately lead to a greater sense of (literal) empowerment.

What we call *voltage* is the force that makes electric currents move, also called the *electromotive force*. The higher the voltage, the stronger the current. In your body, stronger voltage means more energy running through your wires and a brighter inner light. When the amount of voltage flowing through our system drops, we have less energy available to power all the processes in our bodies. Disease and loss of vitality are the eventual results of a low-voltage state.

ELECTRIC BODY, ELECTRIC HEALTH

While scientists have been studying human bioelectricity for over one hundred years, the new technologies and discoveries of the past decade have brought a much fuller picture of our electric bodies to light. Every month, it seems, more studies are published that support and validate the experiential work I've been doing on the body's electromagnetic system—what a team of researchers at the National Institutes of Health in 1994 deemed the "biofield."

Just a few months ago, I was a participant in a first-of-its-kind online summit called the Body Electric, where I gave a presentation on how sound affects our electric health, alongside thirty-six other pioneers who are also considering and working with our electrical nature from other angles. It was thrilling to witness a new way of looking at not just our health but also the world around us, emerging as more and more people begin to "think electrically."

What I have discovered, and what forms the main premise of this book, is that taking care of your electric health is a much easier, more efficient, and even more fun way of approaching health than the standard chemical-mechanical approach. It is more efficient because our electric body is *primary* and *causal,* so working on this level allows us to get right to the root of things. It is the blueprint for our physiology and the template that gives rise to what is occurring in the body. When we get issues sorted out of our electrical systems—primarily resistance and distortion manifesting as pain, uncomfortable emotions, and bad habits—the issues in the physical body take care of themselves. It's an elegant, backdoor kind of solution to what ails us.

In this book, we will talk a lot about how to improve our electric health by raising our voltage. When our voltage is high, we have sufficient "juice" across our cell membranes to keep operations running smoothly and allow us to conduct greater amounts of electrical charge. In a battery, voltage refers to the difference in electric potential (in other words, the difference in electric charge) between the positive and negative terminals. Raising voltage means increasing the electric charge between the positive and negative battery terminals, which makes the battery more powerful. Think about it: A light bulb with a higher voltage shines a brighter light because it has a greater electric potential.

This is essentially what's going on inside your own electrical system. Your body is literally a battery. You are full of salt water, which conducts electricity. All your cell membranes carry a charge. Every organ and system in your body has its own electromagnetic field. I have a little device called an *energy rod,* which is a clear tube with electrodes at either end, and when you hold both electrodes, you complete the circuit and the lights light up and it buzzes. This is a very useful tool for showing people that they are in fact conductors and generators of electricity and that you need a closed circuit for the energy to flow through. It is fun to use in a circle of people holding hands—if one person releases their grip from the person next to them, the circuit gets broken, and the lights and noise stop.

When we recognize our biological systems as rechargeable batteries, we start to think in simple terms of charging versus discharging: Where is your battery meter? What depletes you, and what replenishes you? Where does the meter need to be for you to function optimally? It's easy to tune in to where your battery is; most people know the answer immediately. And most people become aware very quickly that they're discharging far more than they're recharging. Let's check in right now: Ask yourself, on a scale of one to one hundred, where is your personal battery meter? Where would you like it to be?

Have you ever noticed when your phone gets down below 40 percent, the power seems to drop faster? It is the same with our health. There is a point we don't want to dip below because the downhill slope gets faster.

I like to keep myself topped off with close to 100 percent energy, because my performance is best when my energy is high. When my battery starts to drop, I lose focus and effectiveness. I'm not getting good gas mileage, and I'm no longer delivering the output I need to deliver. But when my batteries are charged, my body is strong and healthy, I can get my work done, I can keep my house clean, I can stay resilient in the face of daily stressors, I can take care of my health.

I've worked with thousands of people with chronic illness over the years, and I have come to have a somewhat different perspective on the current epidemic of diseases like Epstein-Barr, Lyme disease, Crohn's, chronic fatigue, fibromyalgia, chronic pain, and so on. I'm asking that you rethink all of that. The bottom line is a low battery. Voltage is low as a consequence of too much resistance blocking the natural, healthy flow of energy in the system. We become like a flashlight with a weak battery and a dim light, without the energy necessary to renew and replenish ourselves.

Having had my hands and forks in the energy fields of thousands of people, I have observed that all these diseases are characterized by low voltage and are the result of insufficient battery power. It's just a lack of energy, of juice. You've discharged and given away more than you've recharged and received. Your cells need a certain amount of electrical charge across their membranes to regenerate themselves. When our bodies have sufficient energy running through them, they fix themselves. When the flow of energy is blocked, our bodies don't have the resources necessary to repair themselves and to return to a natural energy-conserving state of homeostasis. When we return to a state of higher charge, the body's natural healing intelligence directs that energy to where it's needed.

Voltage as pH

I had been studying electricity and the biofield for many years when I discovered the work of Dr. Jerry Tennant. In Tennant's work, I first encountered the idea that *low pH is the same as low voltage.* The "pH as voltage" equation was the keystone that really clicked everything into place for me. When you're looking at health from a chemical perspective, there's only so much you can do to change your pH: You can eat green vegetables, you can detox and cleanse, you can take supplements. But when you look at it from an electromagnetic perspective, there are *so* many things you can do to raise your voltage (we will get into these later in the book).

This means that being religious about eating clean and taking handfuls of supplements isn't the only way to stay healthy and prevent disease. When we look at it from an electrical perspective, we have all these new tools for getting healthy and solving our problems. This is particularly exciting to me as someone who has never been a fan of eating mountains of vegetables.

Dr. Tennant, an ophthalmologist who is also a board-certified practitioner of homeopathic and alternative medicine and author of the book *Healing Is Voltage,* argues that the most critical aspect of healing is the body's ability to make new cells that are able to do their job properly. When our cells go to reproduce themselves, we want the vibrational blueprint to be clear so that they know what they're supposed to be doing and how to do it.

Tennant explains that pH, or voltage, plays a key role in cell regeneration. Over the course of our lives, we're constantly putting wear and tear on our systems, and the way we regenerate ourselves is by making new cells. We're doing this all the time: The lining in your gut is only three weeks old, your skin is six weeks old, and your nervous system is eight months old. We keep ourselves healthy and heal wounds and diseases, first and foremost by making new cells—and it's when we lose this ability that disease and premature aging occur. If our bodies don't have the energy to make new cells, diseased organs won't be able to heal and regenerate themselves. When voltage drops, entropy begins to take place in our bodies due to insufficient juice available to keep everything functioning properly.

Here's where pH comes into play: The body is designed to maintain an optimal balance of acidity and alkalinity, and an optimum voltage of roughly -50 mV (millivolts). Our cells function optimally in a moderately alkaline state, at a pH of between 7.35 and 7.45, and with a cell voltage of -25 mV across our membranes. When a cell is in distress or deteriorating in some way, it needs the body's voltage to be at an optimal level of -50 mV in order for healing to occur, according to Tennant. Also according to Tennant, cells are designed to run at -25 mV (pH of 7.45), but they need -50 mV to make a new cell.

When pH/voltage drops below that, molecules known as *free radicals* start to proliferate. Free radicals are unstable atoms lacking an electron. They arise in low-voltage environments where there isn't enough abundant electrical energy to spread around, and in turn, they create more acidity/low voltage. All toxins are electron stealers, also known as free radicals. Tennant uses the term *electron stealers* because these molecules are missing electrons and are looking to snatch them up from anywhere they can get them—which ends up being our cells! (An *antioxidant,* on the other hand, is a molecule that has excess electrons to give away, which is why they are so good for us.) We *need* electrons for our cells to be able to do their work. When a cell's electrons are stolen, the cell is damaged or destroyed. New studies have shown that cancer cells proliferate, in part, by stealing electricity from the cells around them, which causes further disease and decline.

So when people say that disease occurs in an acidic state, another way to look at this is electrically: What they're really saying is that disease occurs in a low-voltage state where the body becomes weak and electron stealers are running the show, and entropy, dissolution, and poor health are the result.

Tennant, like myself, has observed that the majority of disease begins as an emotional event. Emotions are stored in and around the body as magnetic fields and also as corresponding molecules that have hidden themselves in various places in the body. If you have a bunch of old suppressed emotions that are stored in one of your organs and in some part of your biofield, that's going to create resistance and tension and make it more difficult for electrical flow to pass through. If we want to get healthy, from an electrical perspective, the first order of business is to open an inquiry into the vibrational backlog of emotions that is clogging up our circuits and blocking the natural flow of energy that keeps us healthy and vital.

Emotions and Electric Health

You'll be discovering throughout this book why emotions are the key to electric health. It's often our emotions that kill us—or rather, it's the stress of mismanaged and repressed emotions. In Biofield Tuning, we don't look at any emotions as negative or bad. They're all welcome guests that deserve a say in our lives. This is the single greatest trick to having high voltage: to not judge or suppress any of your emotions but rather to seek to manage them appropriately. It's about learning to understand and master your emotions and allow them to flow through you.

All energy is electromagnetic, it's movement in our being. When we learn to flow with the movement of our emotions, to move with our natural inclinations toward what feels best and appropriate, then we learn to master conservation of energy, which enables us to keep our batteries consistently high. This is not necessarily easy to do. Most of us have been taught to *suppress* rather than *express* our feelings and emotions, and there are limitless means of suppression that our culture provides.

In my observation, this is where many health-conscious people are right now: We're eating the right things, we're drinking the celery juice, we're going to yoga, we're meditating, we're following the self-care rules. But we still feel like crap because we're not paying attention to our emotional health. I spent many years trying this supplement and that supplement and honestly can't say that I ever found anything that made a noticeable difference. I'm not saying that supplements are useless; however, I will say that they were useless for me. I spent a lot of money and piled up a whole bunch of plastic bottles that I then ended up throwing away. I have a friend who has hundreds of supplement bottles in her kitchen cabinets, and none of them have solved her problems, because her problems are rooted in unhealed emotional wounds. They are electromagnetic in nature, and that cannot be fixed with a pill—a chemical solution.

My students and clients consistently say this: "As soon as I started addressing the emotion part of the equation, I started to solve my problems. I started to have more energy. I started to feel better. I started to not be sick anymore." If you've been doing all the right things but you're not where you want to be in your life, this is the next step of the journey: to really understand the emotional territory of your body—which *is* your electromagnetic body—and to work with it.

I recently heard from a woman who stumbled upon Biofield Tuning after seeing the best doctors in the world and doing "absolutely everything" in her power (infrared saunas, juicing, vitamin IVs, acupuncture, and on and on) in an attempt to recover from a serious toxic mold exposure. A Biofield Tuning practitioner whom she worked with helped her to understand that while she had been working from the outside in to get healthy through lots of external interventions, to get back to optimal health, she needed to work from the inside out—healing and releasing her suppressed emotions, working through old traumas and the blocked energy that was the result of those stuck emotions and frozen traumas, so that her body had the inner resources available to heal itself.

Her first tuning sessions triggered a significant emotional release and had the immediate result of making her feel lighter and more energized. As she continued the work, she found that physical pain, as well as fears and anxieties that she had carried for years, simply dissolved. As she stepped into the fullness of who she was, unburdened by the emotional blocks that had stymied her for so long, and with newfound vitality, her impact as a speaker and author also increased.

I am going to talk a lot about Biofield Tuning not to sell you on how great it is (like most approaches, it has its limitations) but because it is the framework I have been operating in that has revealed to me the bigger picture of what I am sharing. When you start managing your emotions better because you understand how they operate in your biofield, you free up huge amounts of energy. While this sounds simple, it is going to take some pages to spell out the finer details of how this works.

Use Your Mind Wisely

In my own life, it wasn't until I started feeling and expressing the things I hadn't been letting myself feel, or didn't even know were buried there, that I started having more energy and being able to solve the problems in my life. It wasn't until I discovered that it was also the things that I was *believing* and *saying* about myself that were having the greatest impact on my well-being and energy levels—and started to change those things—that my life started to go in the direction I wanted it to.

The truth is that our minds can make us sick and they can make us well. The stories we tell ourselves are stronger than any supplement. If you keep saying, "I have this disorder," "I'm broke," "I don't have time," "I'm not creative," and if you are telling yourself that the solution is in something outside of you, you are giving your power away. Your mind created the problem, and your mind can solve the problem.

I had a student in my class a while back who said she had Hashimoto's disease, and I gave her a hard time about that statement. "Who is Hashimoto?" I demanded playfully. "And why do you have his disease?" It made her question what it was she was saying and believing about herself. She went on to turn her whole health situation around by taking control of her story. I barely recognized her the next time I saw her. She looked like a completely different person. When we change our *tune* about ourselves and our lives, our bodies also change.

In certain aboriginal cultures, the elders said that if something wasn't working in your life, it meant that you needed a new story. They believed that you could heal your sickness by getting rid of a bad story and replacing it with a better one. These cultures conceived of the mind as being constructed by all the stories we tell ourselves and others, and I think they were onto something.

One of the biggest things I have learned in my work is how people misuse their mental power in a way that does not serve them—expending their mental energy in stories of victimhood, lack and limitation, or in a vicious inner critic or inner taskmaster. This book will help teach you to use your mind more wisely. My ultimate goal is to help you realize that you can rewire your energetic patterns using your mind alone. In fact, your own mind and intention are the most powerful tools you have for working with your energy system. You are a magnetic being, and you have the ability to impact your magnetic field through the use of your mind.

Here is an example of how I recently applied this process: I am a sensitive person, and one of the things that used to slay me was chemical scents. I couldn't even walk down the detergent aisle of the grocery store. If someone with a heavy perfume sat next to me on a bus or a plane, I actually had to move or I would suffer for the whole journey. One day, it occurred to me that I was playing the role of a victim in these situations and telling myself a story that the offending smells were stronger than I was. So I used my mind to create a different story. I have this big alpaca-wool hat that wicks away snow and cold from my head and does a fabulous job of keeping me warm and snow-free during vicious Vermont winters. I decided to imagine that I had "plasma fur" around my body that could wick away molecules of scent before they even reached me. And it worked! Just imagining that I had an energetic defense allowed me to stride down the detergent aisle unbothered. Ever since I changed my mind about this story, I haven't had a problem. Consider where you are making yourself a victim, when the solution might be as easy as changing your story. Give it a try and see what you notice!

There is one particularly universal story that is at the kernel of almost every dysfunction and problem in our lives: *I'm not worthy.* But that's just a story! It's just words and dissonant waveforms. We want to scrub this and other unbeneficial mental constructs to get back to what I call our *factory settings:* the perfect and harmonious expression of our DNA. When I first started this work, I was astounded to discover that underneath every person's noise was a perfect harmonic signal. There was this rainbow, brilliant song under all the surface-level static. There's a part of us that is not out of sync with the universe but actually quite in sync—beautifully, pleasingly, even jaw-droppingly in sync. We are essentially just stewarding a collection of molecules of creation. You're not part of nature, you *are* nature. The riotous abundance of nature is who you are. The problem is that we can't recognize it because we're so stuck in what Eckhart Tolle calls our *pain body*—the aspect of the self born of the wounds and traumas of a lifetime, as well as the traumas of our ancestors. But no matter how much noise is blocking the signal, I have yet to work on anyone who does not have this underlying template of harmonic perfection.

I love the way Dr. Zach Bush, a triple-board-certified American M.D., describes health as being "fully connected to nature": being in resonance with the essential harmony of that from which we came and to which we shall return. To get back to that place, we'll be going through a process of deconstructing the powerful subconscious programming that makes us feel unworthy, guilty, and "not enough." We're going to deprogram the old stories and beliefs that your mental hard drive has gotten gunked up with, removing the mind viruses that are creating static in the signal and distortion in the field. We'll be bashing through the concepts we've blindly adopted because we don't realize there's another way of looking at things—including questioning notions of "spirituality" that have disembodied and disempowered us. That means digging into the patterns we formed based on our childhoods, our families, our educational and social programming that get us stuck in these lobster pots that we can't get out of.

Raise Your Voltage, Not Your Vibration

An important caveat before we continue: When I talk about raising your voltage, I am talking about something quite different from the popular notion of "raising your vibration."

I prefer not to use the language of "raising vibration." As an explorer of sound, I spend a lot of my time and energy thinking about frequency and vibration. I also spend a lot of time listening closely to people's words—to what they say and the tone of their voice when they're saying it. When I hear people talk about raising their vibrations, what they tend to be referring to is this idea of "ascension." It's the idea that we want to somehow rise above anything ugly, bad, or wrong in ourselves and/or the world around us. We don't want to feel hate or shame, we just want to feel love and good vibes. When we focus our energies on trying to raise our vibrations, what we're doing, perhaps unwittingly, is creating this internal movement of going up and out—out of the body, off the ground, floating up into the cosmos.

Is that really what we want to be doing? People who have experienced trauma tend to cope by disconnecting from their bodies. There's a sense of, *This world is so unpleasant and the pain too much, and I just want to go up, up, and away.* Psychologists call it *dissociation,* and shamans call it *soul loss.* This is the direction we're going when we approach our own healing and growth as a process of raising our vibrations. I've often observed how this way of thinking feeds into spiritual bypassing (or as I call it, *purple-washing*) and point-on-the-horizon thinking. In truth, what we really want to be doing is *descending*—occupying our miraculous and amazing bodies, drawing energy into ourselves from the earth, really committing to being where we are, here and now.

We need to strengthen and be present in our lower energy centers, not just the higher ones that many people tend to focus on when it comes to mindfulness and spirituality. This is where all the juiciness is! We want every part of us to be groovy. We're also going to explore the idea of centering our awareness around our navels and radiating out from our solar plexuses in every direction. As we become lighter and brighter, we become more radiant from the very core of our beings. That's not a high or low thing, that's just a stronger-in-every-direction thing!

On Spaceship Earth, there are no passengers—there is only crew, and we need everyone on board to be sharing their gifts and abilities for the benefit of the whole. We don't need more people with high vibrations and heads in the clouds who aren't picking up the trash in their own neighborhoods. We're in an all-hands-on-deck situation in our world today. We need people here on planet Earth, raising their energy levels and going out and making a difference in the way their souls are directing them to.

And if you'll indulge my inner syntax nerd for just a moment—this hierarchy of high and low vibration is also just incorrect language! When did we decide that higher vibrations are somehow preferable to lower ones? The whole range of frequencies is a part of creation. There are frequencies in the known universe that are unimaginably low. They're light-years across from crest to trough. Why wouldn't you want to associate with those? As far as brain wave frequency goes, the lower the frequency, the more peaceful you are. Monks deep in meditation have extremely low brain wave frequencies, and it's certainly not because they have bad vibes!

When we talk about "low vibrations," what we're really talking about, I think, is a lack of *coherence*. This is a word we'll be coming back to again and again throughout this book, as it is key to understanding the workings of our electromagnetic bodies. What we're describing as low or bad vibrations is really just a chaotic and discordant vibration. It's noise in the signal, an inner symphony that's playing out of tune. From a sound healing perspective, what we want is to *clarify* and *cohere* and *tune* our vibrations. That's what my work is all about: getting the static out of the signal and finding that sweet spot of our own tonal expression.

Sound, as you'll discover, is an invaluable tool in this work: singing, humming, chanting, repeating affirmations, mantras, toning, listening to music. I have often observed a disconnect in our understanding of sound and the electromagnetic body. Many students have asked me why I am talking about electricity so much when my work seems to focus on sound. As you will learn, there's really no separating sound from electricity. Light and sound are both just waves vibrating at different frequencies. Without getting down and dirty into some very complicated (and still poorly understood) physics, the basic idea is very simple: Everything is electric, including your body, and sound directly influences electricity. Sound is nothing more than vibration; it's all part of the electromagnetic spectrum, vibrating at different rates, or frequencies. Vibrations affect vibrations.

What I discovered with my tuning forks is that I could use a vibrating tuning fork as both a magnet and a metronome to modulate and manipulate the rhythms, patterns, and flows of the body's electrical system. This has a direct impact on not just the nervous system but the entire body, because the entire body is transmitting electrical signals. Think about how energized you feel when you're listening to a song that makes you want to get up and dance: that's sound adding energy to your electric body, getting you all pumped up! Sound is constantly affecting how we feel, whether it is the soothing sounds of nature or the cacophony of Times Square.

While I will be providing some sound-based tools, this is not a book about sound healing. If you're interested in learning more about the nature of sound and how it can be used therapeutically, I refer you to my book *Tuning the Human Biofield,* which discusses this in detail.

Effective Problem-Solving: The Key to Good Health

The reason why my practice became successful and the reason why I have been able to move along in the game of life is because I've figured out a hack for solving problems. Thinking electrically is a hack that allows you to level up significantly, because you get to add additional states of matter—plasma and aether—and additional forces of nature—syntropy and levity—to the way you look at, think about, and solve problems. You can solve problems better and faster once you have all these extra tools.

I understand the lobster pots that we unwittingly get ourselves stuck in. I'm a clever lobster, and I figured out how to get out of a lot of pots—an eating disorder, food addiction, chronic pain, digestive woes, financial troubles, marriage troubles, and more besides! But it wasn't through conventional thinking, and it wasn't with conventional self-help. I got them sorted, mostly, through thinking electrically and learning to deal with my emotions.

Sometimes all it takes is looking at things from a different perspective to realize: *Holy crap, solving that problem was easier than I'd thought.* You realize that when your body has enough energy, it has the natural intelligence to direct that energy to the places that need healing. You realize that you have the inner resources to work through whatever challenges you're facing in your life. You have resiliency. You have adaptability. You have clarity. When you increase the signal-to-noise ratio of your electromagnetic body, you're able to hear and act on the voice of inner guidance. You start creating different results in your life without having to muscle your way through things. If your signal is clear enough and your voltage is high enough, your body and life come into a state of flow.

In addition to the information and tools for electric health, including sound, that we'll be exploring throughout the book, there's a basic framework I like to use for solving problems. You can apply this to any of the challenges in your body, mind, emotions, or life, or anything you encounter as you're moving through this book.

Five Steps to Solving Any Problem

1. **Identify the problem.** Clearly recognize, label, and state to yourself what the problem is.

2. **Believe that it's possible to solve the problem.** This is where we often get hung up. I'll get someone to identify a problem that they haven't been able to solve, and I'll say, "Repeat after me: *I believe it's possible to solve this problem.*" When they say that, tension immediately arises in their bodies—revealing all these subconscious places where they don't believe it's possible, which is the biggest reason why they're not solving the problem. You have to get every part of your being on board so that when you say, *I believe it's possible to solve this problem,* the truth of that statement resonates in your body.

3. **Desire it with all your heart.** You have to be absolutely determined to see this through and solve the problem. Stay connected to the feeling of that desire and the *why* behind it.

4. **Believe that the resources you need to solve the problem are at hand.** Because you believe that those resources are available to you, you are able to locate them.

5. **Implement those resources to solve the problem.** Then move on to the next problem!

Throughout the book, whenever you confront a stuck emotion or some old story or programming that you've been stuck in, you can implement this framework to help you work through it. It really works! I did this with my kids all the time when they were growing up. They'd come to me and say, "Mom, I have this problem." I'd say to them, "Well, you're a resourceful person. [I believed in them.] Go figure it out." I would have them go off and track down the resources to solve the problem and then come back and report their findings.

Effective problem-solving is a big key to getting and staying healthy. If you've got a problem, don't just thrash around in it. Don't cry over spilled milk. Be solution-oriented. Figure out a way out of whatever lobster pot you're presently stuck in. Let's just agree right now not to kerfuffle. Kerfuffles lead to a tangled energy field, which attracts and manifests further kerfuffles—it's a vicious cycle that's totally avoidable!

Instead of getting lost in big goals and dreams that feel unattainable, work where you are with what you have. It's tempting to sit around and wish for some kind of quantum leap from point A to point Z, but that's not how the video game of life works. You have to move through each room of each level, and you have to solve the problems as you go to level up. You can't just jump ahead to the good stuff. Know that you have what you need around you right now within the constraints of whatever situation you're in.

JOURNEY OF THE BOOK

Part I, "Thinking Electrically," explores the science of your electric body and the electric universe you live in. We're going to look at the relationship between the electromagnetic energy that powers your human body and travels between the synapses in your brain, the energy that you see in a lightning strike, the energy that powers iPhones and AI, and the energy that powers stars and galaxies. Are they all somehow connected? What we'll begin to discover is that it's all one energy, one electricity, one light. Using the framework of plasma and aether—additional states of matter—we will explore the light within and the light without.

I also share my own story of discovering the biofield and creating Biofield Tuning. I will present my observation of what energy is and how it's working in the body and in the energy field that surrounds the body, as well as in nature. I'm not making any new scientific claims here—many experts in different fields are talking about the same things using their own language. We're just using different words and coming from different angles of approach. We'll gain insight into the electric nature of our biofields—which I have come to see as what we call our *minds*—and how we can start to understand how to better manage the electromagnetic waves of emotions and feelings as they flow through us.

Part II, "Your Biofield Anatomy," offers practical wisdom and tools for working with each of the main energy centers and zones of your biofield. We'll go through each of the major zones in our bodies, exploring their healthy and imbalanced expression, as well as the common energetic patterns and emotional blockages that I have found to be housed there. Using the Biofield Anatomy Map as our guide, we'll walk through the core emotions of each zone, how they get triggered, and what I've found to be healthy and appropriate ways to manage those emotions. I will share tools that I use with my students and clients to help shift the energy from resistance to flow, from noisy to calm, from chaotic to coherent.

This model of the human body and energy system is different from what you may have encountered before, though it shares many features in common with other systems of healing. I do not claim that this framework is carved in stone, only that the observations of the biofield anatomy have proved consistent and reliable. Thousands of other people have worked with this model and map of the energy system and have had similar observations and experiences. I can't say with any certainty that emotions and thought patterns I have mapped in different parts of the biofield are objectively there (future research will allow us to test this); however, I can say that this model has proved useful for myself, my students, and my clients in understanding what ails us—and will hopefully be useful to you!

Part I

Thinking
Electrically

1

My Journey to Discovering Electric Health

For over two decades now, I've been doing something rather weird: I've been using tuning forks to work with the human energy field. In fact, I've used the forks to effectively map the terrain that is the roughly six-foot space around each side of the body, which spiritual traditions call the *aura* and scientists call the *biofield*. A tuning fork is simply an acoustic frequency generator: it's an instrument that can be used to generate a single tone. What I've been doing is using the tuning forks like sonar. I approach a person's body, bounce sound off them, and listen to the signal that comes back. This is the basic premise of Biofield Tuning, which I will explain in greater depth later in this chapter.

What began as a side hobby in my part-time massage practice in 1996 has since morphed into a global organization, with teachers, students, and practitioners and classes worldwide, something I definitely did not anticipate when I picked up and started exploring with my first new set of tuning forks. And what seemed very far-out when I started in a conservative area of Connecticut in the '90s has now become much more commonplace, as sound as a medium for healing has proliferated in both conventional and alternative medicine in the last decade.

It was never my intention to become a "healer" and certainly not to become a "thought leader" in the fields of therapeutic sound and electric health, but my quest to heal myself from the trials of my childhood ended up leading me on a journey of discovery that opened up this entirely new and empowering paradigm of electric health. To be perfectly honest, the *why* that got me into all of this in the first place was sheer vanity and self-interest. That was how it started out, at least. I just wanted to know I could look and feel better.

WHERE THE JOURNEY BEGAN

I grew up as the youngest in a large family, and then, as a consequence of skipping two grades, also became the youngest and littlest at school. Being small and geeky, I was at the bottom of the pecking order every-where I went, and I was picked on and teased a lot. The roughhousing and tickling and Indian rope burns and camel bites, never mind the biting sarcasm, delivered to me by my siblings, who were six to twelve years older than I was, was all in good fun, but it hurt. I was told that I was "too sensitive" and should be more like my sister (who was the same size as the rest of them) and just let it roll off me.

As the runt of the litter, I had zero power to set boundaries, and get-ting emotional about it was met with "Stop your nonsense." Not sur-prisingly, I discovered early on that I could soothe the hurt and console myself with sugar. There is a photo of me around age two and a half lying on the floor of the pantry with an open box of Lucky Charms next to me, and I look like a little stuffed doll, clearly having just eaten myself into a carb coma.

When I turned sixteen, I suddenly stopped being little and geeky. My braces came off, my glasses gave way to contacts, and my Dorothy Ha-mill haircut grew out. Just for the heck of it, I decided to enter the Miss Teen Connecticut pageant. Much to my amazement, I won runner-up (and got a hug from Halle Berry, who was Miss Teen All American that year) as well as the title of Miss Photogenic. This was a game changer. Suddenly, I was pretty. And being pretty meant that you had to be skinny.

The trouble was, I was hopelessly addicted to sugar and carbs. I had managed to starve myself down from my then healthy weight of 132 pounds or so (the weight I am now, actually) down to 125 for the pageant, but I lied and said that I was 115 pounds, which is what I had in my head I needed to get down to. At five foot six and big boned, it was a ridiculous goal to be that skinny. But everywhere I looked, magazines and television and movies all showed me that skinny was beautiful, and I bought it hook, line, and sinker.

At seventeen, I found myself struggling with working in a pizza parlor and caught in between wanting to be skinny and wanting to eat pizza. It started to really mess with my head, and I found myself, much to my teen beauty queen horror, putting on weight. Then one of my coworkers told me that being bulimic worked for her—she could eat what she wanted and never gain weight! So I decided to give it a try, and before I knew it, I was caught in the grips of an incredibly shameful and consuming cycle of bingeing and purging. On the outside, I looked like I had it all together, but on the inside, I was an emotional, compulsive mess.

When I was eighteen, I tried to stop, but I couldn't. This was alarming to me. I couldn't understand why it seemed to be impossible for me to change my own behavior. Every day, I swore I would stop, and then I would find myself throwing up in the bathroom again. *Why the hell can't I stop doing this?*

My mother tried to help by sending me to our new family doctor, but after our session turned into an argument over the nature of reality, he threw up his hands and told me he couldn't help me. Without any other resources available to me, I turned to self-help books. I must have read hundreds of books on psychology, health, spirituality, and human potential, including Wayne Dyer, Deepak Chopra, Marianne Williamson, Tony Robbins, Napoleon Hill, and all kinds of other stuff besides. But I was going from one self-help book to another, bingeing on them like I binged on sugar, and I wasn't finding the miracle that I was looking for.

By the time I turned twenty, many attempts to quit and many self-help books later, I realized two things. One was that I'd been programmed to have an eating disorder. As young women in America, there are two signs that are held up to us. One is "Be skinny," and the other is "Consume."

Women are told that we must be thin and beautiful to be worth anything in this world, and we are also supposed to be good consumers and buy things. I realized that becoming bulimic was the natural way for me to do both: I could consume, and I could be skinny. When it dawned on me that this behavior wasn't necessarily *my fault* but rather was a by-product of the bad inputs and programming I had been subject to, it was a huge relief.

The second thing I realized was that it was my hand and my mouth that were perpetuating this behavior. If I wasn't in control of myself, who was? I realized that I had to take responsibility for my own behavior. Nobody was going to save me. Nobody was going to fix me. It was up to me. This awareness empowered me to finally stop purging, but I couldn't stop bingeing on sugar and carbs. So I started bingeing on exercise, going for two four-mile walks a day, endlessly obsessing about what I was going to eat, when I was going to exercise, and how fat I was. It was the mental drama, more than anything, that bothered me, that I wanted to get free of. I resented how the disorder had hijacked my mind and body, and I struggled mightily to free myself from the grips of it. And gradually, slowly, over the course of many years, I was able to get on top of the problem.

However, it took until I was forty-four years old (with endless books read, courses attended, and dollars spent) to finally conquer that addiction once and for all and get myself to a place where I ate when I was hungry and stopped when I was full and had zero cravings for anything except whatever it was that my body needed. It took me twenty-six years to get where I was trying to get "on Monday" when I was eighteen: to master my relationship with food, as well as fully heal the chronic indigestion, heartburn, stomachaches, and food sensitivities that plagued me for years. And, as I would discover, that required addressing the many hidden pockets of emotion that I had stuffed away and was managing with food.

I had decided to not go to college out of high school and instead saved the money I made at the pizza parlor and a second restaurant job to take a backpacking trip to Europe when I was eighteen to "find myself." I spent eight months traveling by myself, and in that time, I did find myself—in cafés, writing constantly. It became clear to me that I liked cafés and was also inclined toward writing. But my writing at that time was a way to process my guilt over eating two chocolate croissants and ducking into the café bathroom to throw them up, and clearly, getting to writing anything meaningful was going to have to wait.

Shortly after my return stateside, the idea flashed in my mind to open a café in an extra space in a building that my parents had recently bought for their mail-order business—an old carriage barn in a nice corner of town with plenty of parking. It was a perfect location for a restaurant, and we were a family of foodies who always knew we were going to have a restaurant someday, so I didn't have to do much convincing.

In August 1989, my mother, two of my four brothers, and I opened the Vanilla Bean Café (named after my childhood nickname, Bean) in Pomfret, Connecticut. Fortunately, by the time we opened the restaurant, I had cured myself of my bulimia, but being surrounded by sweets and baked goods was like being an alcoholic running a bar. I was working from 6:00 a.m. until after 10:00 almost every night and subsisting almost entirely on coffee, sugar, and bagels.

In the first four years of the restaurant, we grew from 16 to 140 seats, took over the entirety of the building, and beefed up our staff from the four of us to over thirty employees. It was great that it was successful, but it had taken a huge toll on me. Working hundred-hour weeks, constantly on my feet, had just about killed my body. My adrenals were shot, I had gained thirty pounds, and I developed chronic mid-back pain and crippling TMJ that randomly shot shooting pains through my jaw and head.

I was starting to hate people, and I was also starting to hate food. I was exhausted. In 1994, I reached a juncture where I just couldn't take the physical pain and emotional stress of being surrounded by food any longer. I pretty much bailed on the whole scene and left to go to massage therapy school, not because I wanted to be a massage therapist but because it had become clear to me that my real passion lay in figuring out how to be healthy, and I needed a place to start. I also needed to fix my back and my frazzled mental and emotional states.

I had become interested in natural health and considered becoming a naturopath, but I didn't want to go back to school for however many years it would take to get my degree. So I moved to Boston, started attending massage school, and began practicing better self-care. I started doing yoga and eating better, lost weight, and was beginning to finally feel sane and healthy when my mother got a diagnosis of a brain tumor. This brought me back home to Connecticut, where I became my mother's caregiver and stepped back into the restaurant. Sadly, she died within two months of her diagnosis, and I found myself having to fill her very big shoes.

However, I was still determined to carve out time for my health studies, and I began to do a small massage therapy practice on the side while I continued my independent studies on health and healing. In 1996, I read Deepak Chopra's *Quantum Healing,* which introduced me to the idea that everything is vibration. Based on my self-study, I came to subscribe to this notion that we are fundamentally vibration. We're pockets of vibrating energy; we're essentially just waves in space. And if that's what we are, then treating vibration with vibration seemed very logical and elegant to me. I went out and bought every book that I could find on the subject of vibrational medicine, which wasn't too many back then, and that was what brought me to sound. If you are a research junkie like I am, you know that one book always leads to another and to another and another. You just keep on going down endless rabbit holes.

I went down a very big rabbit hole on the subject of sound, and I have yet to emerge from it. No sooner had I finished my initial stack of books on the subject, I received a Gaia catalog in the mail that featured a set of "tuning forks for healing." Intrigued, I ordered them. Each fork was tuned to a different frequency, which the little instruction booklet explained was correlated with the different chakras of the body. The forks were in the C major scale, and the idea was to use C on the root, D on the sacral, E on the solar plexus, and so on up to the crown chakra.

PICKING UP THE FORKS

I started playing with the forks in my massage therapy practice, and right off the bat, I made some surprising observations. I thought that if I activated the C fork above the body, it would just sound like a C. But it didn't. The tone changed depending on where I put it. As I moved the fork around the body, in some places it would go sharp and loud, while in others it would go flat. Sometimes the tone was bright and clear, and other times it sounded full of static. Sometimes the sound would fade out very quickly for no discernable reason. It behaved in a way I didn't anticipate and couldn't predict. (This is a place where skeptics invoke room acoustics and the doppler effect, which do play a role in the changing tones as well. However, after just a bit of exposure to the process, it becomes evident that something else is also going on.)

That was my first big observation: *The forks seemed to be having a conversation with the body.* Whatever kind of noise the body was making, whatever the quality of its acoustic emissions, those waves seemed to be propagating off the body and intersecting with the tones produced by the tuning forks. The forks didn't just provide a one-way input; they created a *dialogue.* As I moved a tuning fork around the body, it changed in pitch and tone and volume and timbre, and that change seemed to be reflective of what was going on in the person's physiology. I discovered that I could change the tone that was being emitted by hanging out in areas that didn't sound right.

In the areas where the tone got loud, I equated that loudness with increased energy. Because I had been working with the chakra system, and because chakras were centers of energy, it made sense to me that it would be louder over the chakras. Then I made this very curious discovery that I could hook into these loud spots and actually move them. I called it *click, drag, and drop.* It was like using a magnet to drag iron filings. In short order, I developed this protocol of finding the loud spots around the body and dragging them into the closest energy center. Then it wouldn't be loud over the left hip anymore, and it would be much louder over the energy center itself.

As an aside: I have never been crazy about using the word *chakra,* because it plays to the division we have between "conventional" and "alternative" approaches to health. Many people have been conditioned to immediately invoke a response of "pseudoscience" when they come across a word like this. In my effort to bridge the divide between science and spirituality, I prefer to use more neutral or familiar language. However, there is no

English equivalent for the word *chakra,* because this feature of our energy anatomies does not exist in our Western conceptual framework, so we will settle for using it in this book. So while I am not a big fan of the term and am not in any way a Vedic scholar, it will have to suffice in the absence of an English equivalent.

I did not begin this work assuming the presence of the chakras, but while exploring the field, I discovered that there really *are* energy centers along the spine at each place that there is a nerve plexus (an area of greater electrical activity) in the physical body. In keeping with the idea of what is called subtle energy being a *higher harmonic* of more tangible energies, it makes sense that there are both physical and nonphysical concentrations of energy in these places. You can think of the subtle energy that spins in a chakra (Sanskrit for "wheel") as a higher harmonic of the electricity that is present in the nerve plexus. And it was clear to me, based on the input that I was getting from the forks, that these chakra points were indeed areas of increased energy.

My next discovery was that I had this very curious ability to understand the noises that the fork would make. If the tone went sharp or flat or fuzzy, I would get this sense of what the sound meant. Often that came in the form of a message that felt as if it were being dropped into a slot in the back of my head—what I've come to think of as my "mail slot." I am not sure where the information that drops in comes from: my higher self, guides, angels, or God itself—who knows!—and I honestly don't mind it being anonymous. Either way, I have learned to recognize and trust these messages when they drop in. Interestingly, this particular area, where the spine joins the skull beneath the occipital ridge, is recognized in some circles as the Alta Major chakra, also known as the "Mouth of God." My jaw dropped to the floor when I first saw this on brain and consciousness researcher Tiffany Barsotti's slide at a conference. "That's my mail slot!" I said to the person next to me.

When I would encounter a distorted sound, I'd feel that little slot open, and a note would drop in and say whatever it was. I would hear a sharp tone around someone's shoulder and say, "It sounds like you have pain here." Inevitably, the person would confirm that they had been dealing with shoulder pain. Then I discovered that if I continued to hold the fork in the area that seemed sharp or atonal, after a little while, the tone would sound clear. People started coming back the next week and saying, "Hey, that pain in my shoulder went away after you did that sound thing. Can you do it again?"

In short order, my massage therapy practice morphed into a sound healing practice, for the simple reason that the sound worked and it was helping people. But I was still only doing this as a hobby, a side gig. This was New England in the mid-'90s, and when I told people I was doing chakra balancing with tuning forks, you can imagine the kind of response I would get. Someone once even told me, "Of all the woo-woo stuff that's out there, what you do seems the *most* woo-woo." Now, this was not what I was going for. I'm about as logical, sensible, and left-brained as they come. I had no interest in being a "healer," and people perceiving me as some kind of airy-fairy, crystal-wearing New Age type was really not what I wanted. I had an image problem, and for that reason, I kept doing my sessions quietly on the side while I continued to work part-time helping my brothers at the restaurant.

In December of 1999, my husband was in a car accident where he was hit at high speed by a drunk driver, and the fallout from this accident and the events that followed had the effect of completely devastating us financially. I won't go into the details, but the upshot is that we ended up selling just about everything we owned and packed our 220-pound English mastiff dog and our boys, who were then one and four years old, into a restored 1971 VW bus and headed to Vermont to start a new life there.

After spending some time working low-paying jobs (mostly all one can find in the beautiful but very rural and poor mountains of Vermont), it occurred to me that if I wanted to get anywhere financially, I was going to have to start another business. My background was in food, so that was the logical place to look. We considered buying a restaurant, but with ruined credit and limited capital, that idea went nowhere. I was doing a few tuning fork sessions here and there, but at that time, I was very clear that I had no desire to make the strange and hard-to-explain practice my primary vocation, even though it continued to be fascinating as a hobby. I finally decided that going into the specialty food market was a good idea, and after spending many Sunday nights walking around grocery stores examining what products were selling and where there might be an unfilled niche, I decided to start making and selling organic kettle corn. At that point, you could get kettle corn at fairs and festivals, where people lined up for the stuff, but not in stores. In all honesty, I had never even tried it, but it struck me as a good idea.

I managed to get a small business loan, bought the equipment, taught myself how to make kettle corn (it is no easy feat to stir a giant kettle while popcorn kernels covered with boiling hot oil and sugar are flying out at you), and started whipping up batches of the sweet-salty snack, which I called Mama's Special Kettle Corn. I made it organic, because that was where market trends were going, and flavored it maple, of course, because we were in Vermont and that seemed like the natural thing to do. I started bringing around samples to local stores, and within a short period, we were supplying over fifty stores, and it was flying off the shelves every week. My grand plan was to grow the business and then sell it to Frito-Lay and retire early. I was moving right along in that direction when something happened with my little sound healing hobby that changed everything.

FINDING THE FIELD

One morning, I was working with a client who was complaining of pain and a sense of pulling in her neck, jaw, and shoulder. She'd been for numerous different kinds of treatments, and nothing had made a difference. She had seen an osteopath, an acupuncturist, and a massage therapist, and nobody was able to help her. I started out the session doing what I usually do, hanging out with my fork in the area near the body part in question, when I heard a loud noise out the window about eight feet away. I stopped what I was doing and went over to the window. I looked out and didn't see anything, and then I turned around and activated the tuning fork as I was walking toward her. And when I got to be around three feet from her body, I suddenly hit a loud spot. When I passed the tuning fork through it, the tone got loud, and then when I was through it, the fork got quiet again. *Wow, that's so strange,* I thought. I had been finding these loud spots over or right around the body, but this one was almost three feet away from her, just hanging out in empty space. *What's up with that?*

I used my click, drag, and drop method to hook into the loud spot and drag it all the way back to her throat chakra and drop it in there. (I had found when I was working on the body that there's a kind of vortex in each of our major centers that sucks the energy in to redistribute it throughout the body—or at least that was the sense I had of what was happening.) The woman went home and called me the next day and said, "Eileen, my pain and that sense of pulling is completely gone."

This was all getting curiouser and curiouser. When my next client came in, I again started around six feet away from the body and began combing inward toward the midline of the body. There was all kinds of stuff going on! All around the body, I was running into walls and channels and eddies and loud spots and nebulous spots. It was an incredibly diverse terrain that I was encountering. I didn't quite know what to make of it.

In these areas where there was a lot of distortion in the sound, there also seemed to be physical "stuff." I would be combing in toward the body with a tuning fork and I would hit something, and it would literally feel like I was moving through molasses.

This energy that I was finding—it had mass and what felt like "charge." There was real *substance* there. And if it were material, I thought, it should be the domain of science, not just spirituality or mysticism. I read as many books as I could on the aura and the human energy field, but it didn't really explain this phenomenon that I was encountering. Instead, I went and tried to find Western physicists to help explain this to me. I looked for scientists to talk to, but none of them would give me the time of day. A sound therapist in Vermont waving tuning forks around people's auras was not of interest to them (go figure).

Then there was also the fact that I could move the "stuff" with the fork and get it to shift from what appeared as being "stuck" in the field around the body to getting back into circulation in the body. Well, that was really weird! It was incredibly mysterious. I had so many questions: *What is this stuff? Has anyone ever measured and named it? And what laws of physics are governing the fact that I can move it with a tuning fork?*

The next thing I discovered was that there were patterns in the field that seemed to recur from one person to another. Much to my surprise, I observed that the same emotions seemed to reside in the same places in each person. For example, I kept observing—or more precisely, hearing— the emotion of sadness in the area off the left shoulder. In person after person, I kept hearing sad stories there, and the client would always confirm them. And then I discovered the angry stories in the area to the right of the liver. Then I started to hear frustrated stories hanging out down by the left hip. There seemed to be this whole vibro-acoustic structure that appeared to exist in the atmosphere around the body.

What soon became clear was that the energetic disturbances I was picking up correlated with the emotional and physical traumas that people had experienced throughout their lives. The energy field seemed to be acting as a record of our life experiences of pain, stress, and trauma from birth onward, with older experiences moving out like rings on a tree. I learned to use the tuning forks like sonar. As the forks were passed through the field, their changing tones reflected changes in the terrain of the biofield. Blockages of flow, static, and distortions were audibly apparent. Different emotions revealed themselves to have different frequency signatures, reflected in the harmonics of the vibrating fork. Fear had a very distinct pulsing quality to it. Guilt, grief, anger, and other emotions all had their own unique signatures and locations in the field.

Reading and translating the information I was finding in the field was like teaching myself braille. Slowly, over time, I decoded the language of vibration. Of many strange things, the strangest part of all this was that there didn't seem to be any precedent for what I was finding. In all the books I'd read, I hadn't come across anything that talked about patterns of information in the human energy field. The human energy field was revealing itself to have a certain anatomical structure to it. It seemed to hold our emotional history, the record of our life experiences, in a very organized way. It was like a very delineated storage system. For a long time, I didn't believe it, because I'd never even heard anything like that before. *If that existed*, I thought, *wouldn't someone have already discovered it?*

But I couldn't deny the patterns I was observing. It was becoming clear to me that our memories, instead of being stored in the brain—or perhaps *in addition* to being stored in the brain—appeared to be stored in this field around the body. The areas of the field on the right and left sides of each chakra appeared to be like file drawers containing records of a specific emotion or state of mind. And I seemed to have this curious ability to uncover these records, dig out the difficult memories, figure out what they were related to and what emotion was involved, and then help my client to reintegrate them into the body.

I continued to question the validity of my findings. Meanwhile, my practice kept getting busier. I was helping people to solve their problems—to get rid of pain, anxiety, disease, even marriage and financial troubles—and they were telling their friends, and their friends started coming to me with their problems. The more people I saw, the more these same patterns showed up.

What happened when I started working out in the field is that, consistently, my therapeutic outcomes became very dramatic. People who had severe anxiety or chronic pain for thirty years would find that their symptoms were gone in one or two sessions. The feedback that I was getting from my clients was unbelievable. It was the kind of transformation that so many people were looking for. It's hard to find things that facilitate that level of transformation. There's a lot of suffering in the world and a lot of things that people use to try to fix it that don't really work. And here I had stumbled into something that was so elegant, so simple, and so effective . . . and yet so weird! It was an odd thing to be using a tuning fork six feet away from someone's body and to be slowly dragging these pockets of energy through empty space.

Then one day, when I was hard at work creating a business plan to automate my popcorn production, a piece of what struck me as "certified mail" was delivered through my mail slot. It said: "The world needs harmony more than it needs another snack food." I got the very clear direction that I needed to go to college, get some degrees, and do academic research so that I could investigate this phenomenon that I was observing and come up with a scientific language and understanding of it. The message came in loud and clear: It was time to sell the kettle corn business so that I could go learn and teach about sound.

I also knew that having a degree would help with the persisting image problem I was having. This work was helping people with their problems, and I felt the need to get it out in a bigger way and to explain it in rational, grounded language to show that this wasn't some woo-woo nonsense. It was real, scientific, and practical. It worked, and there had to be a logical explanation as to why. So I sold the business and enrolled in Northern Vermont University, which was conveniently five minutes from my house and home to one of the only undergraduate degrees in wellness and alternative medicine in the country. I was able to complete my undergraduate and graduate degrees in five years and wrote a master's thesis, "Exploring the Effects of Audible Sound on the Human Body and Its Biofield," which became the basis for my first book, *Tuning the Human Biofield*.

But the real learning came from the thousands of hours I spent with my forks in people's fields, mapping this new landscape of the biofield.

2

Mapping the Human Biofield

Between 2006 and 2010, before and during being at school, I used my tuning forks to map the new terrain of the human energy field. Luckily, I lived in the middle of nowhere in the mountains, and my home office was extremely quiet, which allowed me to listen very closely to the overtones and undertones of the forks. It took several years, but like putting together the pieces of a puzzle, the entire picture of what I now call the Biofield Anatomy Hypothesis gradually emerged.

The Biofield Anatomy Hypothesis is a model of the structure of the mind that my research has revealed over the past twenty-five years. Just like the brain is compartmentalized and different areas are responsible for different things, so are our energy fields. Like neuroscientists have mapped the brain and figured out that different parts of the brain have different functions and correlations, I mapped the biofield. That process led me to discover a particular anatomy of memory storage.

This is my hypothesis, in a nutshell: I believe that the human biofield is a diffuse electromagnetic medium (a *bioplasma*) that surrounds and interpenetrates the body and stores the record of our life experiences. What we call *mind* and *memory* are actually inside this electromagnetic field. The information of everything that we've ever experienced, and even what our ancestors experienced, is encoded in standing wave format in the body's electromagnetic field, with specific areas holding specific types of experiences. In this model, *your body is inside your mind,* rather than the other way around.

Bouncing sound off bodies and listening to the signals that came back revealed a universal pattern that appeared in everyone. Your biofield, like your brain, is compartmentalized, with different emotional experiences stored in different stratospheric locations. Emotional experiences, like memories, are stored in standing waves around the body. Different emotions have different frequency signatures, which is how I'm able to identify them. This isn't rocket science, and I don't have any special abilities for hearing. In fact, I needed years of speech therapy as a kid, and I had to take six years of singing lessons with six different voice teachers (the first five proclaimed me hopelessly tone-deaf) before I could learn to sing on key. If anything, learning to really *hear* has been one of my biggest challenges. But in time, I learned the language of frequency— and eventually, I taught it to others. When I teach this to my students, most everyone can hear it and feel it, and if they don't right away, we find everyone learns it in time. Sadness really does sound like sadness, and fear has a distinct pulsing quality. For some, it can take a little longer, but with enough time and experience, I believe that anyone can learn this language. Especially in a class, an area of sadness is evident to everyone present, the same way that you can recognize a sad song as being sad, even if it has no lyrics.

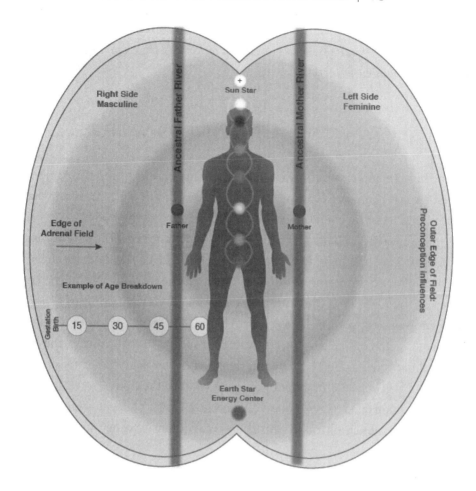

The field is also time lined: The information at the outer edge of the field relates to gestation, birth, and early childhood, what's closest to the body is current or recent, and everything else falls in between. It is defined and contained at the outer boundary by a double-layer plasma membrane located roughly five to six feet away from the body in all directions. As we make our way from the edge of the field in toward the body, we're taking a journey through time from preconception to the present day. What I've been able to do is use the tuning forks like a needle on an album, to read the vibrational record of a person's life. If I were working on a sixty-year-old woman, for instance, and I hit a patch of distortion roughly halfway through the field on the left side of her heart (which holds information related to sadness, grief, and loss), it would likely reveal a heartbreak, divorce, or loss that she went through around the age of thirty.

HOW BIOFIELD TUNING WORKS

The human body is not only an instrument, it is a self-tuning instrument. Just like you can use a tuning fork to tune a piano or a guitar, somewhat miraculously, you can also use a tuning fork to tune the body.

The practice of Biofield Tuning is essentially a process of using tuning forks to scan through the electromagnetic field of the body and find places of dissonance and resistance. Through the introduction of the co-herent sound input of the tuning fork, chaotic waveforms come to a more harmonious expression. They start to be less of a snarl and more of a sine wave. It's almost like ironing out wrinkled sheets. In that process, the energy flow that has been trapped in that part of the field is able to release, and the fork acts as a magnet to drag it back into the body.

States of mind that we habitually energize create patterns of distortion in the field, which ultimately result in breakdowns of order and function in the body.

We know that magnetic fields guide electric currents. By shifting the body's magnetic field and thus shifting the electrical flow in the body, we are able to release pain, tension, stuck emotions, and trauma. Pain is a manifestation of too much current running through the wires, and we can redirect that energy by manipulating the magnetic field. Like Chinese medicine practitioners who do pulse diagnosis, with tuning forks, we are able to sense the rhythms of the currents in the body—which we then shift with the forks, rather than acupuncture needles. I have had many instances of taking someone from an eight or nine on a pain scale of ten down to a one or zero in twenty minutes or less, simply by rearranging the way that energy is flowing through the body.

I think of all these places in the field where we have perturbations and stuck energy as what Eckhart Tolle calls the "pain body." In his book *A New Earth,* Tolle describes it as "the remnants of pain left behind by every strong negative emotion that is not fully faced, accepted, and then let go of, join together to form an energy field that lives in the very cells of your body." The pain body consists of all the suffering and struggle you've been through and the imprint it has left on the way you see yourself and approach your life. When most people refer to themselves, they are referring to their pain body. We identify ourselves with our wounds and create a wounded self-image.

Most of us have had the experience of going through hard times and feeling like a part of ourselves got left behind. As we go through the struggles and stressors of childhood and getting older, bits of ourselves start to fall away. We leave little pieces of ourselves behind. But they don't drift out into the world around us; they actually stay in our own energy field. If you see an older person who's had a hard life, it's almost like they've spilled out. There's a sense of scattering and depletion. The amazing thing about working with tuning forks is that we can find that "stuff" that's spilled out and bring it back and reclaim it. Think of it as entropy versus syntropy. *Entropy* is losing order over time, while *syntropy* is the restoration and creation of order. I think of Biofield Tuning as the syntropic process of bringing lost life force back into our bodies.

On some level, we will always be indelibly imprinted with our life experiences, but we can release the emotional charge and consequently their hold over the present moment. You don't have to be living in the patterns created by growing up with an alcoholic father or a cycle of abuse. Working in the field allows us to discharge or unplug the pain body, and then plug back into our neutral center, returning to the now, and reconnecting to nature. Instead of reacting inappropriately based on all the information in the field, getting triggered, and repeating the same old patterns, we are able to respond with a clear mind in the present moment.

It struck me once that what we were doing was very similar to the shamanic concept of soul retrieval. This process is premised on the idea that when a person undergoes a traumatic experience that they don't have the wherewithal to process in the moment, a bit of their soul breaks off and stays in a place where it is unavailable to the person. It's the work of a shaman to use their active imagination through a process called *journeying* to go back in time and space, find the soul fragment, retrieve it, and bring it back to the person. The shaman will actually blow or physically place the soul fragment back into the body. When I learned of this process, I was astounded by how much Biofield Tuning sounded like sonic soul retrieval! We're finding these lost pieces of self and bringing them back into the body, into circulation and availability.

Not only in shamanism but also in Western psychology do we find this idea that the psyche can become fragmented through trauma and stress—and that psychological health can be restored through a process of reintegrating these repressed and split off parts of self. From a psychotherapeutic perspective, when we integrate the parts of ourselves that we have denied, shut off, and relegated to the shadows of the unconscious, we return to a state of emotional and psychological health. From both the shamanic and the Western psychological perspective, as well as the perspective of Biofield Tuning, healing is a process of restoring wholeness.

The way that we restore wholeness, from an electromagnetic perspective, is by bringing these fragments of frozen light, of forgotten self, back into circulation and availability. People who have had a lot of trauma learn to live with fewer and fewer parts of themselves on line. When they start to reintegrate these lost parts of self, they can achieve what feels like superhero status.

These fragments are our hidden potential! I often liken them to the concept of Easter eggs in a video game. They're these secret pockets of gifts and potential that you find as you're moving through the game. When you find and claim an Easter egg, you're literally increasing your electrical power. With more bioavailable energy at your disposal, you get more done. You become a better manifestor and a stronger player in the game of life.

Using the language of sound, we can describe this phenomenon in terms of coherence and incoherence. When you are in a coherent state, it means that all the vibrational patterns in your system are in phase with each other. That's what the word *coherent* means: "in phase." If something is coherent, it hangs together. It's unified and harmonious. In the human energy system, coherence is a state of conservation of energy. An incoherent state is one in which there is a lot of stray, unintegrated frequency formations in our conscious minds and our bodies. If you've got a lot of things in different phases in your system—that divorce you never dealt with, that alcoholic father, that fifth-grade teacher who traumatized you—you will experience some degree of incoherence. When people have experienced a lot of trauma, they have all these bits of energy stuck out in their field, and they're resonating at many different frequencies.

Essentially, our inner orchestra is either making music—all the different players and frequencies within ourselves are coming into phase to play a harmonized, unified tune—or we're out of phase and making noise: something is flat here, something is too fast there, something's not even playing somewhere else. Coherence is when that inner orchestra is brought in tune, in its right rhythm and proper flow, into that *sweet spot* of harmonic perfection. As we find these out-of-phase pockets and harmonize them, we become more integrated and energized.

PATTERNS OF MIND

I can literally read your mind with a tuning fork, because everything in your mind is a vibrational pattern in your energy field. I can tell you if you had a head injury when you were five, I can tell you about the personality of your mom and your dad, I can find the age of that divorce or job loss, because all that information is encoded in this vibrational language in your field. But I can also find the mind frames that you regularly inhabit, the core beliefs you hold about yourself and life, and the stories you repeatedly tell yourself because they also show up as patterns in your biofield.

It's not just traumas and suppressed emotions that we find in the field but also mental patterns and belief systems. After having my hands and forks in the energy fields of thousands of people, I've observed many common patterns of mind: the shared tonal expressions of the stories we tell ourselves, the thoughts we loop in, and the beliefs we hold.

Beliefs aren't just in our minds, they're in our energetic makeups. They're actual structures, like energetic lenses. It's like when you go to the eye doctor and they flip all these different lenses over. Some make your vision clear, and some make it cloudy. The lenses affect how we see things. So beliefs are like lenses within our biofields that our perception of reality gets filtered through. If you believe that you always lose things and you're looking for your keys through that lens, they might be right in front of you but you won't see them. They're in your blind spot, and it's because you have this belief, this story, this charge around losing things that's distorting your vision. Or if you interpret someone as a villain, you're going to put that spin on everything they say and do to back up them being a villain. That's what you're going to see.

Everyone has these patterns that they act out over and over again. The tracks that get laid down early in life become the grooves we get stuck in. Although an infinite potential exists in every moment, we continue to choose what is familiar to us, what fits in with our beliefs, what is moving along the track that was already laid down before we were even aware of what was going on. This is how we get stuck in life: Over time, patterns of belief and thought redirect our energies into tangles and whirlpools, and these vibrational patterns then turn into patterns of behavior that create patterns of results.

The phrase that *believing is seeing* is actually truer than *seeing is believing*. We filter our experiences of reality based on the lenses of these beliefs, and in many cases, they don't serve us. Let's take baby boomers as an example. I have found individuals of the baby boomer generation have very similar patterns in their fields from the birthing and child-rearing practices they were subjected to. Most people of this generation were left to cry it out, and they were bottle-fed formula on a schedule. These are very damaging patterns that can lead to a chronic frustration over unmet needs and a lifelong pattern of speaking but not being heard (as well as sugar addiction due to the sugary nature of formula). If you were bottle-fed on a schedule as a baby and every time you cried and asked for food you were ignored, you weren't held, you weren't given food—you're going to form a belief that it doesn't matter what you say, because people don't listen to you. That belief is going to affect the tone of the language you use. If you're speaking and not being heard, it's because your tone is infused with that belief and people are responding to that belief, so it's all a reinforcing process. *See? Nobody listens to me. I was right.* But that's just a story. If you shift that story and that pattern, and you start honoring your own truth and listening to yourself, then people listen to you. The actual tone of your voice changes, carrying the information that you are worthy of being heard. We shift our whole experience of life by shifting these lenses.

The baby boomer pattern is a nonlocalized pattern that can be found in different locations across the field, impacting many different systems, organs, and parts of the body. Other patterns are more localized. As an example of a localized pattern, let's take a look at two extremely common patterns that show up in the hips—a loaded area of the biofield that holds many undigested emotions and dysfunctional patterns of thought and behavior.

For instance, it's very common for people to have pain and other issues in the right hip, and I've treated many clients complaining of these issues. What I have found, almost without exception, is that people with right hip issues have a pattern of compulsive overdoing. They're constantly in motion: constantly thinking, doing, go, go, go. Typically, this kind of overthinking and overdoing is driven by feelings of guilt and inadequacy. What they do is start running all their energy in a spinning wheel in the field off the right hip. I have yet to meet someone with a right hip replacement who did not have this pattern.

Shifting over to the left side of the field, we find the pattern that I refer to as *posture of victimhood*. This pattern is concentrated around the bottom of the left hip in the field off the root and sacral chakras. Our energies tend to congregate there when we're habitually telling ourselves stories of powerlessness and blame and when we are spinning in frustration over unmet needs and frustrated non-doing. This is what the energy feels like: *spinning*. It's like a whirlpool in the field that traps huge amounts of life force.

This pattern of victimization often ends up zigzagging throughout the body. It can go over to the liver, and we can have a hot, angry response there. It can come into the left side of the heart, and we can have a sad, hurt response. It can go up to the right side of the third eye if we're dwelling on the past and continuing to feel victimized by something that happened to us. It's just a zigzagging pattern of imbalance in which our energies are really off the center midline.

The first time I noticed the posture of victimhood as a distinct pattern in the field was many years ago when I was working on an individual who had a tremendous amount of energy stuck in his field and shockingly little in his body. He was suffering from low energy, poor digestion, and an inability to fully engage with life. What I found in his field was a lot of stories—and stories that the person was very attached to! Many of these were angry stories of victimhood. It was easy to see why his digestion was suffering: All his inner fire was tied up in unexpressed anger over these perceived injustices. There is a tremendous amount that I can say about this particular topic, because we all suffer from it to some degree. We'll come back to it in Part II.

It's interesting to note that the number of hip (and knee) replacements in the United States has skyrocketed, and they are now becoming more common on much younger adults than in the past. It's no mystery to me why that is! Any time something starts to go south in some part of the body, there's an issue in the vibrational template, in the blueprint of our physiologies. It's the emotion or state of mind underlying that part of your body that is causing the problem. When you're in this imbalanced state of overthinking and overdoing, all that energy and light that's supposed to be in your right hip is actually being siphoned off into the field. That light is supposed to be giving order, structure, and function to your cells, tissues, and organs. When it spills out to the right of where it's supposed to be, when it becomes imbalanced, that part of your blueprint is missing. As the body goes to repair its cells, it can't read the blueprint and fix the problem because that information and energy is not present. So the physiology starts to break down. What we do in Biofield Tuning is find the energy that's spinning out there, neutralize the vibrational pattern it is stuck in, pick up the energy with the fork and with our intention, and then guide it back into the body where it belongs.

At one point when I had particularly bad mid-back pain, I trained my two boys, who were then six and nine years old, so that they could work on me. When I asked my six-year-old to summarize what was going on in the process, he said, "We're taking energy from where it doesn't belong and bringing it back to where it does belong, so it can get to work doing what it is supposed to do." In all the years that this work has been conducted, I would say that is one of the very best definitions of Biofield Tuning!

ENERGENETICS: THE TONE OF THE SONG OF OUR DNA

After I decided to fully commit to tuning, I got an office in the downtown of the tiny village of Johnson, Vermont (population circa 3,600). I had no sign on my door, and yet, people would find their way to me for healing. Person after person walked into my office and declared, "I'm here to heal my ancestral lineage," or "Can you help me clean up my genetics?" I didn't know how they found me, but I would always tell them that they had come to the right place. When we work with the template of the biofield, we're able to go beyond our own personal histories, because the standing waves that are present in the field contain not only our own life histories but also the tonal histories of our ancestors.

An important feature of the biofield anatomy is what I call the *ancestral river,* located around ten inches off the body on both the right and left sides. It's impossible to mistake this zone when you hit it, as the tone is markedly different from the relatively consistent base tone of the individual that permeates the rest of the field. I call it a river because that's literally what it feels like. There's a strong current of energy flow. I am speculating here, but what I have concluded based on thousands of hours of clinical practice is that the left side holds the DNA information related to maternal lineage and the right holds genetic information from the paternal line.

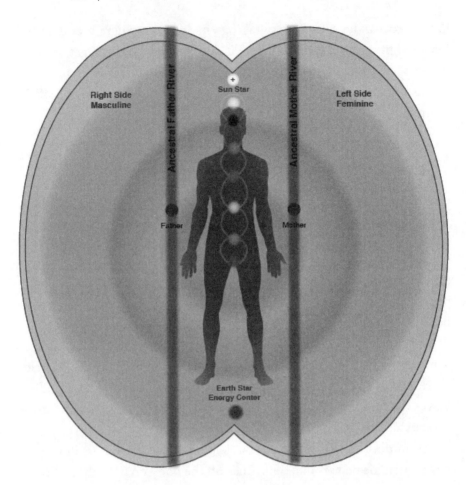

This area holds your inherited genetic as well as *energenetic* information, as I call it. Energenetics is *the tone of the song of our DNA*. We don't just inherit hair color and eye color. We also inherit all the emotional experiences and tonal qualities of our ancestors.

It became clear to me early on in my practice that babies are not clean slates. We come into this world preloaded with all kinds of programming and noise. We come in with depression, anxiety, blockages around money, a predisposition for addiction. The tonal patterns of these imbalances have already been set. I've seen people have the tone of depression in the record of their fields going back to birth—and it turns out that their moms or dads had depression, and they inherited that tonal expression. It creates an undertone of depression in the body's inner symphony. I've worked with many people with depression who have tried, unsuccessfully, to treat it at the level of *me* and *mine* without realizing that the roots often go much deeper than just them.

DNA is as much vibrational as it is chemical. We carry the music of our ancestors, but we can actually change the key that our inner songs are written in, even if they've been playing a certain way for generations. Working in the biofield, we have an opportunity to go into our vibrational templates to clean the chalkboards that we inherited and rewrite the music of our DNA. When we stick a fork in the ancestral river and introduce a coherent frequency, it serves to clarify the tonal expression of those who came before us.

The influence of energenetics is one of the most powerful discoveries I have made in this work. Ancestral influence and intergenerational trauma are a huge part of health and well-being that have largely been ignored, although in the last few years, more and more research has shown just how affected we are by the difficulties of those who came before us. American culture is so heavily individualized and future-focused that we have blinders on when it comes to the influence of those who came before us. We've been programmed to leave the old country behind, so to speak, and focus on becoming the self-made man or woman. But what we fail to account for is how difficult it is to self-actualize when you are carrying around a set of traumas, emotions, and limiting beliefs that are not your own.

We go through life blaming ourselves for having these dysfunctional patterns and then feeling guilty and inadequate for not being able to change them. But it's not necessarily easy to shift the DNA files that got corrupted way before we came along and then were passed down the line. Using our own awareness and intention, using sound and other healing modalities, we can work with our vibrational templates to scrub those inputs and get back to our factory settings, but it's a process that requires some patience.

It tends to be a relief for people to realize that it's not their fault that they inherited these patterns from Mom and Dad. That information is just in the DNA stream that is informing the sound current that informed the shape and expression of who you are—and it doesn't have to be a life sentence. I encourage you to keep this in mind as you're reading this book and exploring the patterns in your own field. Know that what you're dealing with may not have originated with you. Consider that it may not be your fault! You just popped into the space-time continuum and inherited a whole lot of anxiety and depression and crap to clean up. It's you, but it's not just you. It's your parents and their parents and the cultures they lived in and the whole human story. Looking at our own habits and struggles, we have to ask ourselves, "How many generations back does this go?" If you start to look at it in terms of "*the* problem" instead of "*my* problem," it can make it much easier to process and solve.

I have seen many times that any changes that we make go downstream to those who come after us. When we change the tonal quality of our own DNA, it's not just influencing our ancestors but also our descendants. I've had many clients over the years tell me that as they shift and they heal and they clarify their signals, they would notice that their parents or their children start to shift as well.

A WORKING SYSTEM AND AN EVOLVING HYPOTHESIS

I want to stress that this is a working model. The biofield anatomy and the way that I've defined these regions within the biofield are a hypothesis. It is my own subjective discovery, so I'm not going to call it fact. But I call it a working model, because it has proven useful, replicable, and reliable in both detecting and correcting imbalances in the electromagnetic field of the body. My students and clients regularly tell me how stunned they are at how accurate the model is, particularly the time-lined element. Biofield Tuning (and the Biofield Anatomy Hypothesis, on which it is premised) is a model that seems to work.

Exploring the biofield with sound has, and continues to be, a journey of discovery. I have explored the composition and structure of the biofield through my clinical practice, while researching my master's degree, and later, through continued research with organizations like the Consciousness and Healing Initiative (CHI) and the Institute of Noetic Sciences

(IONS). In collaboration with scientists at IONS and CHI, I'm using the scientific method to investigate this hypothesis from a variety of angles—stay tuned for the findings! I have years of research ahead of me, with other experts, to really understand the biofield on a scientific level.

What I wrote in *Tuning the Human Biofield* remains true today: I have more questions than answers and still consider myself more of a student than an expert in this field. Until science provides us with a more objective understanding of what I've found here, we are engaged in the work of hypothesizing.

However, that electricity is the juice that makes us run isn't up for debate. And it doesn't just run our bodies, as we will see—it runs the whole show going on around us as well. My attempts to make sense of my unusual observations quickly led me beyond the body—and then even beyond the world of solid, liquid, and gas. When you step into this world of energy and the biofield, you step into a world of plasma. You step into a world that includes the forgotten concept of aether. We're going to venture into that world to discover a new understanding of ourselves and our environment that is alive, connected, and full of light.

3

Electric Universe, Electric You

One of the things that makes Biofield Tuning rather difficult to explain is that it encompasses two additional states of matter beyond solid, liquid, and gas. These are plasma—the fourth state of matter that is proven and scientifically accepted—and a hypothetical fifth state of matter, the aether, that has been the subject of scientific debate for centuries. We're going to explore in depth what these states of matter are, how they together comprise our electromagnetic environment, and why they are directly relevant to our experiences of everyday life. And remember: We are still talking about energy, electromagnetism, and electricity—we're just getting more specific with our language and grounding our understanding of energy in an exploration of the *vehicles* of its transmission.

Why does this matter? Is it just empty intellectualizing? It matters because when we widen our perspective on the nature of reality and "the way things are," we change the possibilities and opportunities that are available to us. The real magic and abundance of life is in its *interconnectivity,* and that connectivity is happening, from my perspective, through the mediums of plasma and aether. We can tap into this collective electromagnetic field and find support and possibilities and energy and potential there.

COSMOLOGY: THE BIG PICTURE

But before we get into plasma and aether, let's zoom out and take a look at our larger cosmological story. Cosmology is the overarching story of life itself, the assumptions about reality that we rarely question. The discovery of a different cosmological story was the discovery that changed everything for me.

Our current cultural, secular big bang cosmology goes something like this: In the beginning, there was nothing, which for no reason suddenly exploded one day. After it exploded, for no particular reason, it achieved a high degree of order. Ever since then, entropy (dissipation, dissolution) has been the dominant force. This clockwork space, which is winding down, is full of mysterious dark energy and dark matter. Space is an empty, cold vacuum. No one can hear you because sound doesn't travel through space, and besides, we're probably the only ones here, out in this meaningless corner of our galaxy. Gravity pulls us down, and entropy rips us apart.

This is a very dark, heavy, disconnected, and even sad view of the whole thing! But what is important to understand is that this worldview came into being before we had Hubble and other incredible technologies that could really feel and see into space—and whose findings have begun to paint a very different picture of what's going on in the cosmos. Our cosmological story, it would seem, is evolving.

Scientists are now finding that space is electric and that our sun, rather than being an isolated thermonuclear furnace that is constantly burning itself out, is electrically connected through plasma to the rest of the electric universe. We are discovering that space isn't empty after all—it is filled with plasma of varying densities and formations. And sound waves travel through plasma! They are called Alfvén waves. Plasma forms ribbons, and sound travels through these ribbons that connect galaxies.

And as it turns out, entropy isn't the only game in town. Syntropy (also called *negative entropy* or *negentropy*) also exists! Even though we observe the descent into chaos in space and the world around us, we also observe the continual arising of order. Levity is also a thing! Gravity isn't just a force pulling us downward. We now know that sound waves fall upward, that there is actually a force of nature that goes up, not just down. There is abundant evidence that sound has been and can be used for levitating objects. Try listening to some calypso music on steel drums—you can feel the levity in your body!

From this perspective, the universe is a living, connected, electrical organism, made up of all the light we can and cannot see, continually changing its shape and expression as entropy and syntropy do their continual dance of destruction and creation. And we are part of that illuminated, eternal, mind-boggling amazingness!

PLASMA: THE FOURTH STATE OF MATTER

Let's learn a little more about plasma—the state of matter that you most likely never learned about in school.

It's a curious thing that many people have never heard of plasma, which comprises as much as 99.99 percent of the known universe, according to some sources. Plasma is defined as the fourth state of matter. It consists of a gas of ions—atoms that have some of their orbital electrons removed—and free electrons. Electrons and ions are free-floating, which means that the gas is electrically conductive and responds strongly to electromagnetic fields.

Our other three known states of matter all arise from, or more technically condense from, plasma. This "unorganized material; elementary matter" (*Webster's*, 1913 edition) condenses into gas, which condenses into liquid, which condenses into solid, but everything begins as plasma (well, technically, in my humble opinion, aether gives rise to plasma, but we will get to that later). The way plasma behaves informs the way physical matter forms. Plasma is all around us. The environment that we live in is full of plasma. We live in a fluid, electromagnetic environment. When you breathe in, you are breathing in plasma. You are breathing in air that is full of electricity and life. When you're breathing in coastal ocean air that's full of lots of airborne charge, what we call *negative ions,* you're breathing in even more plasma.

Space is made up of plasma! Nebulas are a plasma. Lightning is a plasma. Solar wind is a plasma. The northern lights are a plasma. A Tesla globe is a plasma. We live in a plasma environment. We don't just breathe in oxygen, we breathe in electricity, too! Each oxygen molecule carries four free electrons, which bind to the iron in the hemoglobin of our blood and are then dropped off at cells, providing the body with a constant flow of electrical juice.

Water is a plasma, as Dr. Gerald Pollack proposes in *The Fourth Phase of Water,* meaning that water is electromagnetic. Our blood and all the fluids in our bodies are electrically charged. The electrified water in our bodies actually forms a gel state, the degree of charge present informing how DNA gets expressed. Fire is a plasma. NASA scientists are finally talking about plasma in space after years of referring to it as "hot gas." Stanford and other Ivy League universities have plasma physics labs. We rely on medical innovations that use plasma. Cold plasmas have shown great promise for disinfection. Plasma is a growth market at the moment—if investing is your thing, consider finding an industry that's utilizing plasma (and there are a lot now) and putting your money there!

The sun that heats the earth is made up of plasma. Solar wind isn't just a hot gas; it's a stream of electrically charged particles (plasma!) that's hitting the earth's uppermost part of the atmosphere, the magnetosphere, that buffers this energy and distributes it around the outer boundary of our planet's atmosphere. This isn't new or radical information. Kristian Birkeland, a Norwegian scientist who studied the northern lights, postulated this theory in the early 1900s and was nominated for seven Nobel Prizes (although he was ridiculed until the proof actually came in).

I recently read an article from *Scientific American,* published in 1965, that said the following: "Since 1958 direct measurements of the outer reaches of the earth's field by means of artificial satellites and rocket probes have convinced many geophysicists that the simple picture of that magnetic field must be drastically revised. Far from being free of external influences, the *geomagnetic field is continuously buffeted by a 'wind' of electrically charged particles emanating from the sun,* distorted by electric currents circulating in the radiation belts that girdle the earth" [emphasis mine]. Scientists have known about electric current in space for a long time, but somehow it has never quite made it into our worldview!

Continual planetwide lightning strikes discharge and ground this energy. Space is an electrical environment that's filled with plasma. In some places, it's very diffuse, and in others, like stars, it becomes very dense. Voyager 2, Hubble, and other space probes have been providing us with lots of information about plasma in the last decade. In 2018, the Voyager 2 space probe moved through the equivalent of our magnetosphere—the sun's heliosphere. It actually slowed down as it traversed this wall of "dense, hot plasma" that creates the outer boundary of the plasma bubble that contains our solar system. A report of Voyager 2 observations published in the journal *Nature Astronomy* revealed this fiery wall to be up to 89,000 degrees Fahrenheit.

The plasma that is the stuff of the stars is also what makes up these human systems of ours! Remember, it is the same electricity of the sun and lightning that is powering the electric device that is used to jumpstart our electric hearts when they stop. My hypothesis is that the human biofield is also a plasma, and more specifically, a bioplasma. What is a bioplasma? It's the diffuse magnetic fluid around any living thing, defined by a double-layer plasma membrane at its outer boundary. These living fields were described by Yale professor Harold Saxton Burr as *L-fields,* and he studied them extensively in the '40s and '50s, with various devices set up around the Yale campus. The idea that all life-forms have a living field around them is nothing new; however, many of us have heard that there is no such thing as a field. But as we will see, that assertion goes against observation and basic laws of physics.

Like anything in nature, electromagnetic fields tend to behave fractally. What they are on one level of scale, they are on other levels of scale—as above, so below. This is the macrocosm and the microcosm. The human biofield and our magnetic fields are like a fractal rendering of the earth's

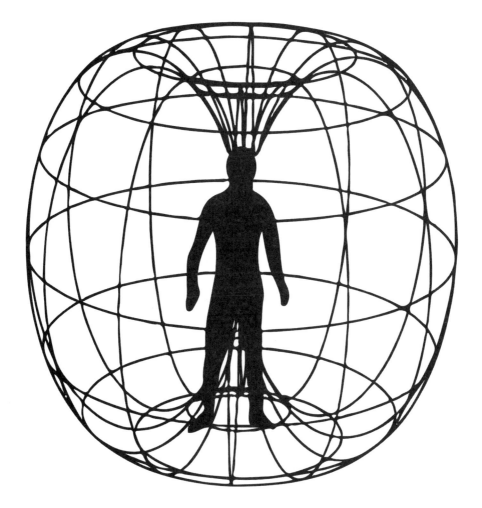

magnetosphere and the sun's heliosphere. There's a double-layer plasma membrane at the outer boundary that protects the organism. In the human biofield, that outer boundary creates the dynamic standing waves that hold information in the field. Just like Voyager 1 and 2 slowed down as they went through the heliosphere due to the resistance caused by a greater density of energy, our tuning forks also can perceive this density at the outer boundary of the field. The waves bounce off the inner boundary of electrical charge, in the same way radio waves bounce off the inner boundary of the ionosphere. Every cell and organ in the body has its own field in addition to being part of the group field of the human body.

For many of you, this may be the first time you have ever heard of plasma. Why is it most of us never learned about this important and ubiquitous state of matter—one that is accepted and studied by Harvard and Stanford scientists? While the concept of the aether has been actively dismissed and allegedly debunked, plasma, it seems to me, has simply been ignored. We know it exists; we just haven't found a place for it in our larger cosmological framework.

Let's take a look at a different cosmological framework—one that acknowledges plasma and its place in our universe.

THE ELECTRIC UNIVERSE

My discovery of electric universe (EU) theory opened my eyes wide to a logical, elegant electrical explanation of the universe and to the work of the early researchers of plasma cosmology. The idea that what is going on in space is all electric and electrically connected is not new. It's just been ignored and sidelined in favor of mathematical equations over observation and experimentation.

Fundamentally, plasma cosmology observes that electricity, which is orders of magnitude stronger than gravity, is what is really running the scene up there. Dark energy and dark matter (mysterious forces that purportedly both hold the universe together and pull it apart) have never been observed—they are mathematical constructs plugged into a mathematical theory of a gravity-driven universe because the electric force is missing from the equations of current cosmology, according to EU proponents. When you look at what is observed in space through an electric lens, it doesn't require having faith in invisible dark forces. From a plasma cosmology perspective, galaxies spin because that is how electricity behaves, not because of black holes sucking from the inside and dark energy pushing from the outside. Over the last few years, the SAFIRE lab has tested the premise of an electric sun and has been able to create a working plasma model in their lab. The University of Wisconsin has also successfully modeled an electric sun and electric solar wind in the lab. This is because plasma is scalable and fractal and behaves the same way whether it is "a star in a jar" or a star in space. This is opposed to the standard thermonuclear fusion model of the sun that has never been successfully created in a lab.

When I started doing research on plasma in 2010, there wasn't much on it to be found in the media or popular press. NASA photographs called nebulas "hot gas." No one raised their hands at my talks when I asked them if they had heard of plasma. But over the last few years, a tremendous amount of research on plasma and more broadly on the electrical nature of all of life, from the subterranean to the astronomical, from the ocean floor to solar wind, has begun to emerge. Incredible work is being done at world-class plasma physics labs at Princeton and Stanford, and an increasing number of studies published in reputable journals are revealing the electrical nature of all of life. We now know that electric currents are found throughout nature, and according to geophysicists, they run the show in space.

Here's some other exciting new evidence of the electromagnetic nature of our terrestrial and inter-terrestrial environment:

- **The moon:** Recent science has shown that the moon is electric. In 2018, for the first time, they detected the presence of a weak layer of charged particles known as an *ionosphere,* roughly one million times more nebulous than the earth's ionosphere. They also found that the electrical activity of the moon is enhanced when it's full. The electrical activity of the moon is theoretically connected through plasma and aether to the electrical activity of our own bodies. Could this enhanced lunar electrical activity explain why more babies are born (as with both my babies), more deaths occur, more psychiatric episodes and emergency room visits are recorded, and more people are arrested at the full moon? There is more charge and more energy in the environment.
- **Bacteria:** In recent years, scientists have identified electroactive microbes that build power grid–like networks, transmitting electricity through the ground. "Not to sound too crazy, but we have an electric planet," one of the study's authors, Duquesne University microbiologist John Stolz, told *The New York Times.* The *Times*

noted that the abundance of electroactive microbes in different ecosystems may support biodiversity and help regulate the chemistry of oceans, land, and atmosphere. The bacteria in our gut are also electric, making digestion an electrical fermentation process.

- **Soil:** In 2017, Cornell researchers discovered high-definition electron pathways in soil—fueled by the microorganisms that live in the dirt and require electrons for everything they do. This seems to spur plant growth. Johannes Lehmann, a professor of soil science who was involved in the study, said, "We've learned the electrons are channeled through soil very efficiently in a high-performing way." Electro-agriculture—supplying plants with more electric current from wires in the ground—is a growing field and has been shown to create higher yields of crops.

- **Bees:** Researchers have identified a weak electrostatic field that arises between a flower and a bee, playing part in an electrical interaction that's critical to the pollination process. Flowers have a slightly negative electric charge, which attracts the positively charged bees, a 2013 study revealed.

- **Birds:** Birds navigate the earth via electromagnetic fields. There is a protein in their eyes, which is also involved in circadian rhythms, that allows them to "see" the earth's magnetic field and use it to guide their migrational paths. Other animals, including dolphins, turtles, butterflies (and yes, humans!), are also known to be guided by magnetic fields—which may be informed by the presence of magnetite in the tissues of all animals. We'll dig into this more later in the book.

- **Human reproduction:** And since we're talking about the birds and the bees, let's talk about sex, too! Research has shown that sex is electric—there is a flash of light when a sperm enters an egg. Orgasms involve an intense burst of electrical activity in the nervous system, vagus nerve, and brain—a literal moment of illumination. As Regina Nuzzo wrote in the *Los Angeles Times*, "In an orgasm orchestra, the genitalia may be the instruments, but the central nervous system is the conductor."

These myriad natural sources of electricity may provide the keys to the future of our species and the planet. Based on what science is beginning to reveal, solar power may be only scratching the surface of what's possible. Scientists across the globe are currently investigating how to harness electricity from bacteria, the atmosphere, the earth's core, and other elements of the environment as potential energy solutions. There is a wealth of innovation and creative solutions to the world's problems just waiting to be discovered in this largely untapped natural resource.

Additionally, many increasingly popular researchers and thinkers, such as Dr. Jack Kruse, Dr. Dietrich Klinghardt, M.D., Ph.D., Dr. James Oschman, Dr. Gerald Pollack, Dr. Claude Swanson, Lynne McTaggart, Dave Asprey, Dr. Zach Bush, and many others are telling the same story from different angles about what I call *electric health*. The topic is lighting up across the globe. At the same time, the conversation about aether is also starting to present itself again, and there are a great many scientists and researchers who are working to bring back this fundamentally unifying and illuminating substrata of creation. Stay with me here. Soon, you'll see how understanding these elusive and fascinating substances called *plasma* and *aether* will directly and powerfully transform your understanding of your own body, health, and life.

4

AETHER:
The Hidden Dimension

All perceptible matter comes from a primary substance, or tenuity beyond conception, filling all space, the akasha or luminiferous ether, which is acted upon by the life giving Prana or creative force, calling into existence, in never-ending cycles all things and phenomena. The primary substance, thrown into infinitesimal whirls of prodigious velocity, becomes gross matter; the force subsiding, the motion ceases and matter disappears, reverting to the primary substance.

—Nikola Tesla

Imagine for just a moment that you are living in a light-filled universe. Connect to the biological light within your body, all the way down to your bones, and the light emanating from your biofield. Feel that your biological system is powered by the light of the sun and stars. Then start to expand your awareness from the light within to the light beyond. Imagine that every living thing—from animals and plants to soil and bacteria to the wind and rain—is alive and dancing with electrical charge. Like a fish in water, you are swimming at all times in an invisible sea of light. The air you breathe and the space all around you isn't empty; it is a medium connected by invisible webs of energy, full of charged particles and magnetic fields. Everything you see, hear, feel, taste, and smell is a part of this sea of light that connects and permeates all things. In your own inner illumination, connected to the "one light" of the universe, you are in alignment with all of nature. Who you are is one cell of light in the universal light body—one note in the cosmic symphony.

For thousands of years, spiritual traditions have spoken of the light of God that fills the universe. But there was also a time, not so long ago, that physicists understood the cosmos as a vast and infinite web of light. Scientists like Nikola Tesla and Albert Einstein used to have a word for the connecting, all-pervading medium of light that gives rise to all things: the aether. Nikola Tesla, a pioneer of electrical science, described the "luminiferous ether" as an ocean of clear light through which all waves travel and the field of infinite potential (the *unified field* or *zero-point field*, in contemporary terminology) that all of life unfolds in.

The aether has a long and storied history in human cosmology. It's universal in almost all spiritual traditions and ancient cultures; it's been hotly contested by physicists for years; and it was alternately rejected and championed by Einstein himself. The story of the aether's removal from science, and its dawning comeback, offers a hidden key to understanding our electric bodies—and the electric universe that is our home.

The contemporary scientific perspective on aether is well illustrated in this quote from an October 2019 article in *New Scientist* with the headline "Einstein Killed the Aether. Now the Idea Is Back to Save Relativity": "As far as dead ideas go, the luminiferous aether is among the deadest. Over a century ago, it picked a fight with Einstein's theory of relativity and lost. Few victories in modern physics have been so total. Today, relativity offers us our best picture of the large-scale structure of the universe. It is a byword for human achievement and scientific progress. The aether, if it gets mentioned at all, is an embarrassing footnote in its rise to glory."

However, as we will see, aether hasn't gone away that easily—and right now, we may just be witnessing its resurrection.

I offer the following information in service of giving you a better understanding of your own electric body. But before we get into the meat of how you can use this information in Part II, we need to lay a framework for understanding the medium we are working in. For this reason, it is worth taking a bit more time to better understand what aether is and how it operates so we have a better sense of our own aetheric makeup.

THE AETHER: A BRIEF HISTORY

Please note: this word is correctly spelled both ways, aether and ether—I use both spellings here depending on the context.

What is the aether? There are many definitions from the lenses of many different belief systems and quite a few strong opinions! For our purposes, we will define the aether as the hypothetical fifth state of matter, but more accurately, it is the primary state of matter that gives rise to all other states of matter. *Aether* is another word for what you're more likely to have heard described as the "unified field" (or just "the field") that, in varying densities and arrangements, composes the things we see as well as the space between them. The simplest definition describes aether as an ocean of clear light that electromagnetic waves arise in, travel through, and dissolve back into. It is the source of all energy, the medium through which the "word" (vibration) gave rise to light. Aether is dielectric, meaning it has the ability to polarize itself into what we call *positive* and *negative charges*, and through torsion—the spiraling dance of those forces—it spins itself into plasma, and plasma spins itself into gases, and then liquids and solids. Matter precipitates from the finest form, aether, and spirals into visible light and then into the density of the physical matter we see all around us. What this points to is the notion that everything is fundamentally aether, woven through different vibrating arrangements into greater and greater density.

In religious terms, *ether* is another word for the heavens, the celestial realms. It is described in many cultures as being synonymous with spirit or God. In many ancient and medieval civilizations, aether was considered one of the elements: the element of *space*. In physics, ether is defined as "an all-pervading, infinitely elastic, massless medium formerly postulated as the medium of propagation of electromagnetic waves." (Note the *formerly* in the scientific definition of the aether—we'll get into this momentarily.) Early explorers of electricity such as Tesla, James Clerk Maxwell, and J. J. Thomson understood aether as the medium through which light traveled.

In the ancient Vedic texts, aether, or space (*akasha*), is said to *give rise to all vibration,* which then creates the phenomenon of sound. Vedic cosmology describes sound and aether as inseparable—and suggests that the aether is the medium through which both sound and light waves travel. It's also believed in the Vedic tradition that aether is the substance that the mind is made of. According to the California College of Ayurveda, "Ether represents the substratum upon which thoughts and emotions ride like waves upon the ocean." The aether and the *akasha* are both seen as holding the vibrational information of everything that ever is, was, or will ever be: all our experiences, thoughts, memories, and emotions. It is the Akashic records—the vibrational "book of life" that holds our individual histories and the history of the collective, in past, present, and future time.

Nikola Tesla, the pioneer of the electrical science that informs so much of the world around us, described aether elegantly as the "primary substance . . . filling all space" in the quote at the beginning of this chapter. In the late 1800s, Tesla spoke of a universe that was electrified, a system filled with energy, underlaid by a universal field that gave rise to all matter. In Tesla's mind, electricity was responsible for all phenomena in the cosmos. Tesla's thinking was deeply influenced by his friendship and intellectual partnership with the Indian yogi Swami Vivekananda, who had been spreading the philosophy of yoga and Vedanta in the West. Fusing together his Western scientific framework and Vedic metaphysical language, Tesla's electric cosmology brought together the worlds of East and West, science and spirit.

All the way up to the turn of the twentieth century, the aether was part and parcel to our understanding of reality. Physicists understood the aether as the medium through which light waves traveled, just the same way waves travel through water. Then, in the early 1900s, the theory of aether was allegedly debunked when it was replaced with the hypothesis of space as an empty vacuum, purportedly in support of Einstein's theory of relativity. Without getting too deep into some very complex science, the short story is that relativity created a framework for understanding space-time that did not require the presence of the aether. Compounding matters was the 1887 Michelson-Morley experiment, which allegedly failed to detect the presence of an aether when attempting to determine whether the hypothetical "aether drag" had any impact on the speed of light. Despite its many flaws, this experiment is routinely cited, along with relativity theory, as conclusive evidence that the aether does not exist.

Another nail in aether's coffin was Einstein's famous 1905 paper on special relativity, in which he dismissed it as "superfluous." And yet, the question of the aether dogged him for many more years. As Einstein's thinking evolved, he became increasingly convinced that there *must* be some electromagnetic medium in space. By 1920, he seemed to have completely changed his tune. He said in an address on the subject at the Leiden University: "More careful reflection teaches us, however, that the special theory of relativity does not compel us to deny ether." Einstein's 1920 statement is worth quoting at length, as it succinctly describes the apparent conflict between ether and relativity:

> *To deny ether is ultimately to assume that empty space has no physical qualities whatever. The fundamental facts of mechanics do not harmonize with this view. . . . The conception of the ether has again acquired an intelligible content, although this content differs widely from that of the ether of the mechanical wave theory of light. . . . According to the general theory of relativity, space is endowed with physical qualities; in this sense, there exists an ether.* Space without ether is unthinkable; for in such space there not only would be no propagation of light, but also no possibility of existence for standards of space and time *[emphasis mine]*.

Well into the 1930s, Einstein toiled to develop a unified field theory that would include time and space as a part of some kind of unified field, which he began to refer to as the "new ether." In his 1938 book *The Evolution of Physics,* Einstein wrote: "[Ether]'s story, by no means finished, is continued by the relativity theory."

By this time, Einstein had publicly recanted his earlier declaration of the aether's nonexistence. But the damage had already been done, and by then, nobody wanted anything to do with the aether. The theory was declared dead—that is, until very recently. Today, mainstream physicists are beginning to reconsider the aether as the theory of relativity reveals more and more pressing structural flaws—suggesting that it may not be the final stop in the journey of our understanding of the universe. Relativity has not been able to explain the forces of dark energy and dark matter. And perhaps even more pressingly, physicists have yet to find a "quantum theory of relativity" that explains how the universe behaves at the smallest scale.

Now, as *New Science* notes, "the key to relativity's salvation could lie in the aether." The article goes on to explain that a small group of researchers since the early 2000s have claimed that aether could have the power to unify physics. And in 2018, two research groups suggested that the aether could provide an explanation for dark energy and dark matter. As further research unfolds in the coming years and decades, we may just see our cosmological story changing before our eyes.

A prominent contemporary defender of the aether is Frank Wilczek, a distinguished professor of physics at MIT who won the Nobel Prize in Physics in 2004 for work he did as a twenty-one-year-old graduate student. Wilczek makes a strong case for a new version of the aether—the "primary world-stuff" that he refers to as *the Grid*—in his excellent 2008 book *The Lightness of Being.* (I highly recommend this book to those interested in exploring the topic further.) In his book, Wilczek presents a number of arguments in favor of a field underlying all of time and space. He describes the Grid as a kind of "cosmic superconductor" (a superconductor is a material that offers no resistance to electrical currents) that powers the rest of the universe. In other words, it is a medium through which electromagnetic waves travel freely.

"We draw power for appliances, lights and computers from the electric grid," Wilczek writes. "The physical world of appearance draws its power, in general, from the Grid."

Even as scientists dismissed the concept of the aether or were ridiculed if they pursued it or incorporated it into their work, the search for explanations for the subtle energetic field that seems to pervade all matter has continued. They've called it by names like the *zero-point field,* the *quantum field,* the *Higgs field.* If you look up the definition of each of these concepts, they sound a whole heck of a lot like the aether. Here is the definition of the Higgs field: "The Higgs field is a field of energy that is thought to exist in every region of the universe that gives rise to and interacts with matter." Since he couldn't call it *aether* because that idea was deader than dead, Peter Higgs named it after himself! Noted physicist Lawrence Krauss wrote that the Higgs field "validates the notion that seemingly empty space may contain the seeds of our existence."

Last summer, I went to an event with Nassim Haramein and his organization, the Resonance Science Foundation, and learned that since Nassim is a physicist, he can't use the word *aether,* but when he is talking about the *quantum vacuum,* he is talking about essentially the same thing. What I found notable at this event was that practically all the presenters were speaking about aether in some capacity, albeit using other language to describe it.

SACRED GEOMETRY AND YOUR AETHERIC BODY

There is a pattern in the heavens, where those who want to can see it, and establish it in their own minds.

—SOCRATES

Also present within the aether is geometry. Everything in nature has a very fundamental geometry to it, from atoms and cells to seashells and plants to stars, planets, and the universe as a whole. On every scale, everything in nature conforms to one or more sacred geometric shapes.

What we call *sacred geometry* is an ancient science exploring the energy patterns through which the universe organizes itself. Why *sacred*? Because they speak to the hidden order, the self-organizing principle, that underlies all of creation. When we attune ourselves to this fundamental aspect of creation, we come into powerful contact with the harmony inherent in the natural world.

This geometry is the underlying architectural blueprint of creation, and as such, it is an integral component of the aether. The aether arranges itself into basic geometric wave patterns—the five Platonic solids—as it spins itself into matter. The Platonic solids are shapes in which all the faces and all the edges are the same size. There are only five of them, and they all fit within a sphere. Twenty-five hundred years ago—before mathematics became secularized—Plato wrote that the physical world was constructed from these shapes.

The repetitive patterns of the Platonic solids that fit into each other and can be scaled to any size are what we call *fractals*. If you've ever looked at a Romanesco broccoli, a fern, or a snowflake, you've seen fractals at work. According to Dan Winter, founder of the San Graal School of Sacred Geometry, the fractal patterns that shape the atom also shape our planets, stars, and entire galaxies.

Our bodies are electrical waves informed by geometry. The human ear mirrors the spirals found at every scale of creation, from galaxies to seashells. The human body is built on what Renaissance artists called the *divine proportion*—also known as *phi* or the *golden ratio*. On a subtler level, our electromagnetic bodies are also geometric in nature. I recently created a set of weighted tuning forks that are tuned to the eleventh (89 Hz) and twelfth (144 Hz) positions in the Fibonacci sequence. When you divide these numbers, you get the phi ratio. I use these particular frequencies to induce the geometric information of the natural harmonics of the unfolding of nature, in perfect proportion. The effect is one of being able to rest more in the ordered geometry that underlies the composition of the human body. The way I understand it is that these frequencies help bring order to our etheric bodies—our geometric templates. One user described them as creating a sense of a "bright inner order."

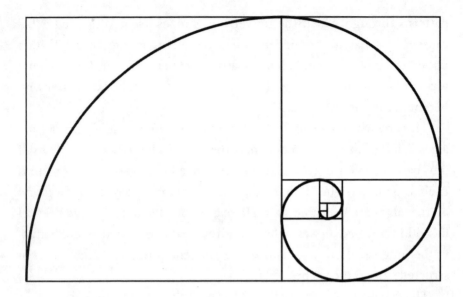

When you avail yourself of these fundamental building blocks of life, something shifts in your psyche. You start to see life from a different lens—one that recognizes a magnificent underlying order and intelligence in all of creation. To truly grasp our own innate beauty and harmony as a part of creation, a knowledge of sacred geometry is an important part of the equation.

Let's take a closer look at two fundamental shapes of the aether: the spiral and the sphere. Since the time of the ancient Greeks, the aether has been described as moving in torsion, or spirals. The spiral is the purest form of moving energy. The universe moves and transforms in spirals, never straight lines. These spiral patterns can be found throughout nature, from snail shells to entire galaxies. As folk musician John Hartford said, "The whole universe is based on rhythms. Everything happens in circles, in spirals."

The sphere is another fundamental form of aether. Tesla and others believed that light and sound waves propagate both spherically and spirally, rather than in the 2D longitudinal and transverse form in which they are typically depicted. While we don't *really* understand the nature of waves, by one view, waves are geometric, patterned information that inform the medium that they're moving through. This is very evident when one looks at the effects of sound waves on water in a device called a *cymascope*, which you can see in videos on YouTube.

What happens when you bring the sphere and the spiral together? You get a *torus*—the shape of the human biofield, the earth's magnetosphere and the sun's heliosphere, and in other forms throughout nature on the macro- and microscale. Some physicists have even hypothesized that the universe as a whole is structured in this doughnutlike shape— mirroring esoteric and indigenous views of the universe as a "world tree" with a central axis and wide-spreading branches and roots. It's been suggested that the torus is a self-organizing, self-sustaining geometric form that optimizes energy efficiency, as it creates a vortex of energy flow up and down the rotating axis. It makes sense that our bodies, and larger planetary bodies, would be organizing in such an energy-efficient manner.

Esoteric traditions describe the physical human body as having an aetheric template, in the shape of a torus, that channels aetheric energies into increasingly dense and charged energies and ultimately matter, all the way down to our bones, the densest part of the physical body. Healing modalities that work with the subtle energy of the body, like Biofield Tuning, directly target the aetheric body—the vibrational template of our physiology—to create changes in the physical body. From what I can tell, aether is the finest form of subtle energy. Within the human energy system, everything from the finest aether to a diffuse plasma is what we call *subtle energy*.

It's my belief that in Biofield Tuning, we are working with the mediums of the aether and plasma. The space within and around us isn't empty; it is filled with light, information, energy, and sound. That's how I am able to uncover detailed information from the record of the person's life history—experiences, emotions, patterns of thought and belief—in the roughly six-foot space around the body that we call the biofield. The aether has the property of holding information and memory, like water does. It's the same thing, in my opinion, as the *akasha* or the Akashic records. In our own aetheric bodies lie our personal Akashic records.

The biofield, as I see it, is both aetheric and bioplasmic. Our bioplasmic, electromagnetic energy field sits in the larger structure of the aether, which condenses from its finest and most diffuse form into the relatively denser bioplasma.

It is through our aetheric bodies that we are connected to all that is. Although the torus shape of the electromagnetic body, or biofield, is marked by a double-layer plasma membrane that acts as its outer boundary, it exists within and is connected to the universal aetheric body. This is how we are all connected, at all times, to everything else in the universe. Our consciousness is nonlocal and part of this vibrating electromagnetic soup of the aether.

BEYOND QUANTUM: RESONANCE IN THE AETHER

The aether is also described as operating holographically, meaning that the whole is present in every part. It is this property that allows for instantaneous communication through any amount of time or distance, explaining things like remote viewing, telepathy, synchronicities, distance healing, and other psi phenomena that have been widely studied and replicated in the lab, despite their woo-woo connotations. It also explains the universe as a connected unit, in touch with and orchestrating all events as a unified whole. Wal Thornhill describes energy as "the movement of matter in relationship to all matter in the universe."

Aether physics offers a particularly elegant explanation for the way distance healing works. I did not believe in the beginning that conducting Biofield Tuning sessions at a distance was possible. In fact, I arrogantly and snidely dismissed it as ridiculous and preposterous. But when I actually tried it, I discovered, much to my amazement, that it was in fact possible, and I had to admit that I had been wrong. I was able to read and modulate the field of my client three thousand miles away (who had twisted my arm to give it a try) in the exact same way I could if someone were on my table. Thousands of students and practitioners have since made the same discovery. The outcomes are consistent: the practitioner can feel and hear and read the person's energy field, and the receiver often has a sense of energy moving and then a subsequent state change. The process works. The hypothesis has been tested endlessly and produces consistent results. Therefore, there must be a natural law that governs the fact that it works.

The way I explain it to people is this: When I do a distance session on someone, I pluck that person's file out of the aether and work on the file, which acts as a kind of hologram for the physical body. Shaping the aether in this way is what intention and manifestation are all about. It's about causing the electromagnetic fluid that is life to respawn to the electromagnetism of our intentions. As quantum theory has revealed, the observer affects the observed. Simply by witnessing and participating in life, we are co-creating it. There is no objective observer in science. Simply by observing reality, we affect the way the ocean of pure potentiality that is the ether condenses into form. The electromagnetism of the mind is affecting the subtle energy of the aether. It's also called a *quantum wave collapse*. Waves rearrange themselves into particle form to match the frequency of our intentions. (If you're interested in learning more about the science of intention, and how it can impact the physical world, I recommend Dean Radin's book *Real Magic: Ancient Wisdom, Modern Science, and a Guide to the Secret Power of the Universe*.)

The notion of quantum entanglement—or what Einstein called *spooky action at a distance*—is also poking in the direction of how distance healing works. But in quantum theory, there's still this idea, in most people's minds, of a vacuum in the middle. There's no *connecting medium* in the popular perception of quantum physics. We are still faced with the problem of isolated particles moving in nothingness, traveling in the void of empty space. But when we bring the aether into the equation, the spookiness is gone, because the medium of connection is present.

I avoid referencing the quantum physics model in my work, and there are a few reasons for that. The first is that quantum physicists tend to get bees in their bonnets when New Age healers and folks waving around tuning forks talk about quantum this and quantum that. Another is that the word *quantum* has several different meanings, and there are many different ways to interpret quantum theory. It's evident to me that we haven't yet reached consensus on how to use these terms. And then there is that famous quote: "If you think you understand quantum physics, you don't understand quantum physics."

But more fundamentally, there's something missing in quantum theory that I believe the aether helps us to resolve. Quantum theory, in my view, doesn't step back and use clear language to offer an elegant explanation of things. It doesn't answer the questions! It doesn't solve the problems. It points toward a connected universe but doesn't offer any sort of medium of connection. There's still this idea of space as an empty vacuum and this mysterious resonance of particles in the void of nothingness, communicated from light-years away. No matter how much I studied quantum theory, I never felt like it was giving me the answers I was looking for.

We know that everything is vibration. Here, I would like to offer a parallel perspective on the idea of "everything is vibration" that is somewhat different from the quantum model. I would argue that *everything is resonance in the aether.* Sound, light, electricity, matter: it's all waves in the aether, resonating at different frequencies.

This diverges somewhat from the standard physics model, which tells us that sound and light are both waves, but fundamentally different kinds. In the standard physics model, what we call sound is defined as a mechanical wave that requires a medium—such as solid, liquid, or gas—to pass through. What we call electricity, however, is an electromagnetic wave that *does not* need a medium—it can pass through the vacuum of empty space. So by this definition, sound is not a part of the electromagnetic spectrum, because it requires a medium, like air or water, to travel through, whereas other electromagnetic waves can travel through empty space. But what if space isn't the empty vacuum we believe it to be? And what if what we call sound is, as many assert, part of the electromagnetic spectrum? Then the whole divide between sound and light dissolves! It's all just resonance, the movement of waves of infinite frequencies and arrangement, in the aether.

In my opinion, there's fundamentally no difference between what we call *sound waves* and what we call *electromagnetic (light) waves*. For one thing, there are two definitions of sound. One is waves in the range of 20–20,000 Hz, within the range of human hearing. The second definition is propagating waves of any frequency. Whether we call it *light* or whether we call it *sound* or whether we call it *electricity,* we are talking about the same thing: propagating waves of different frequencies and patterns. We are taught that sound and light make different kinds of waves, sound being longitudinal and light being transverse. And yet whenever a sound wave is depicted in 2D, it is always shown as a transverse, sine wave. That in and of itself is confusing. To make things a little more complicated, another way to consider wave propagation is that all vibrations radiate spherically, spirally, and geometrically from their source. Take the sun, for example—it is continually in flux, sending out a wide spectrum of waves, from the very low that we would call *sound* to the frequencies of visible and invisible light.

By this view, the electromagnetic spectrum goes from sound to ultra-sound to infrared light, so it's a total continuum of light. Sound is part of the electromagnetic spectrum—meaning that sound and light are both fundamentally electrical in nature. What we call sound—20–20,000 Hz—are waves in the range of what we can hear with our ears. It's a vibration, a wave moving through space, through the medium of the aether. Yes, it needs a medium, but in the model we've been discussing, so does light. In essence: Sound is audible light, and light is visible sound. Sound is really just a lower octave of visible light, or in other words, light is a higher octave of sound.

Sound is electromagnetic! The aether ties it all together and helps to show that sound is a continuum of light. We divide everything and turn all the pieces into nouns, but that's not what's going on. It's just a continuum. Our division has to do with our organs of perception, not to do with what's actually out there. Light is just a higher harmonic of sound, sound is just a lower harmonic of light. It's all waves, and it's all waves through the medium of the ether. Tesla and his compatriots understood it this way, but this understanding just got buried and pushed aside as the aether was replaced by relativity.

"Light cannot be anything else but a longitudinal disturbance in the ether, involving alternate compressions and rarefactions," Tesla said. "In other words, light can be nothing else than a sound wave in the ether."

What this shows, on a practical level, is the role of sound in our electromagnetic health. Sound is a big part of raising our voltages, whether it's the sound of our own voices that we hear in our minds or whether we're breathing with an audible exhale or a sound of pleasure. Sound is electric, it is magnetic, it carries mass. A vibrating tuning fork is an electromagnetic phenomenon. The motion of a vibrating tuning fork produces a weak electromagnetic charge, which is how I'm able to use it like a magnet within the weak magnetic field of the body. When I bring sound into a place that's heavy and stuck, sound breaks that energy up and liberates the electrical flow. When I introduce that into your body, you feel lighter and more lifted and more energetic because of that electromagnetic input.

EVERYTHING IS ILLUMINATED

When we bring aether and plasma back into the equation, we start to tell ourselves a very different story about who we are, where we're from, and where we're going.

This new way of looking at life, the universe, and our bodies runs counter to what most of us were taught in school—and to the thoughts most of us walk around with in our heads about the nature of reality. I am not asking you to believe it, but I am asking you to consider it. This is simply what makes sense to me based on my own research and experience, and to the thousands of people already exposed to my work who all say, "This makes sense," when they learn about it. Examine your own cosmological story and your assumptions about reality, and find what rings true for you.

After I came to really grasp the implications of an electrically connected universe, I never picked up another self-help book again. I had no idea that my journey as a seeker, spending decades sifting through vast amounts of information looking for truth and light, would reach its natural conclusion with the unveiling of a completely different cosmological story. All that time, I had no idea that it was the subconscious cosmological story of darkness and entropy that was continually "harshing my Zen" in the back of my mind. Once I really came to understand the *science* behind "all is one" and "one light," it was as if all this discomfort that had kept driving me to find answers suddenly just went away.

That said, at this moment in time, we don't have conclusive evidence to describe any theory of the universe as absolute truth. And perhaps we never will! Here I cite the brilliant biochemist writer Isaac Asimov: "I believe that scientific knowledge has fractal properties, that no matter how much we learn, whatever is left, however small it may seem, is just as infinitely complex as the whole was to start with. That, I think, is the secret of the Universe."

The universe may just be one great unknowable mystery, far too vast and complex for our puny human minds to possibly comprehend. And whether you believe in flat earth, round earth, hollow earth, expanding earth, or that this is all some kind of matrix simulation, I think we can all agree on the word that Tesla favored: *realm.* When we look at the increasing amounts of evidence mounting around us, it is clear that this realm has at its basis the force we call *electricity.* Life itself is the movement of waves. Light, sound, music, electricity are all movements, spiraling dances, in the aether.

Again, this is *practical* knowledge. Raising your voltage isn't just about connecting to your own electromagnetic body. It's about connecting to the universal electromagnetic body as well—and using that connection to help you become healthier and happier, more resonant, and in tune with all of life.

We can work creatively with the laws of nature to make things happen. We can tap into our own personal Akashic records to better understand ourselves and to change the way we operate. We can enter into a dynamic collaboration with all of life through the connective medium of the aether. It's an incredibly creative and connected landscape we're in. We can have a lot of fun with it if we understand better how it works, which gives us more resources to play the game better. We can work directly with our own aetheric templates to change our physiologies and get back to our vibrational blueprints.

5

Body of Light

Who you are is a radiant light body. That's not some kind of vague spiritual concept, it's a biological fact. You are living, breathing, and thinking right now thanks to the constant transmission of electrical information throughout your system. Your cells literally emit light. The neurons in your brain create a network of light that looks like networks of stars in faraway galaxies.

This notion of your light body isn't esoteric, it's electromagnetic. Without electricity, you wouldn't be reading this right now. Not because your lights or your computer wouldn't turn on but because your *brain* wouldn't turn on. At every moment, tiny electrical impulses are traveling through your entire body, controlling and regulating everything you do: walking, eating, dancing, sleeping, dreaming. It's all happening thanks to the information conveyed by the transmission of these electrical impulses, which travel to and from the brain to nerve branches extending throughout the body, all the way down to the tips of your fingers and toes.

Scientists and medical doctors have studied and documented the body's electrical systems, and this knowledge has been used for many decades to inform their research and treatments. However, while most of us know the bits and pieces, many of us have yet to connect all the dots to see just how much electricity informs and shapes our bodies and minds.

You likely know, for starters, that your brain and nervous system operate on electricity. Doctors can monitor the electrical activity of your brain using an EEG machine, which records brain waves—synchronized electrical impulses from groups of neurons communicating with one another. The frequency of these waves (alpha, gamma, theta . . .) are what determine whether your mind is alert or calm, waking or sleeping, focused or wandering.

Your heart is the other major center of electrical activity in your body. The heart is an electrically driven oscillator that maintains the rhythm of your entire organism. An electrocardiogram, or EKG, monitors the electrical activity of your heart, and a pacemaker regulates it. In fact, the heart's electric field is approximately sixty times greater in amplitude than that of the brain, according to research from the HeartMath Institute. And the electric field of the heart is deeply impacted by our emotions, which are electromagnetic waveforms. As HeartMath cofounder Howard Martin explains:

> The electrical energy produced by the heart radiates outside the body
> into space. The heart's field is not static. It changes, depending on what
> we are feeling. For example, when we are feeling emotions like anger or
> frustration, the frequencies in the field become chaotic and disordered.
> On the other hand, when we are experiencing emotions like compassion,
> care, appreciation or love, the frequencies in the field become more
> ordered and coherent. In a sense, through the electromagnetic field
> created by the heart we are literally broadcasting our emotions like
> radio waves.

Let's not stop there. Your muscles, your fascia, your entire collagen microfiber network are electrical semiconductors. Even the densest part of your being, your bones, are piezoelectric crystalline structures that make electricity when they're compressed, which happens whenever you dance or run or move around. Your blood carries an electric charge. Panasonic is currently exploring how human blood could be used to power electrical devices by conducting research on how blood breaks down sugars to generate energy.

Your body is also comprised of up to 60 percent water (and by some accounts, more), which conducts sound and electricity. In fact, the salt water in our bodies (made up of roughly 0.6 percent salt content) may be one of the main vehicles for the transmission of electricity throughout the body. But the water found in your body is different from the salt water that's in the ocean. In *The Fourth Phase of Water,* Gerald Pollack shows that structured water molecules can arrange into a gel made of ordered, helical structures with an enhanced ability to conduct electricity. This fourth phase of water, also called *structured water,* is the basis of biological life. All the water in our bodies is this fourth state of water. It appears that this highly ordered, crystalline form of water forms intricate networks through which electrical energy flows through the body.

The building blocks of your electrical body are your cells, which were designed to generate and conduct electricity. There is an optimum range of voltage across your cell membranes. The electrical signaling of your cells makes everything happen in your body (an important point that we'll come back to later in the chapter). The bacteria living in your gut are electrical beings, too! Scientists have found that hundreds of different strains of the microorganisms that inhabit our intestinal tracts (both the friendly ones and the not-so-friendly ones) are *electrogenic,* meaning that they can produce electricity—up to one hundred thousand electrons per second per cell. Digestion is actually a process of *electric* fermentation, as we will later explore in greater depth.

You get the idea: Your entire body is a battery. You were designed to conduct and run on electricity, and every part of you carries an electrical charge.

But beyond the nervous system, brain, heart, cells, and other parts of our physical organism where electricity is known to exist, there is also the field of energy within and around your body—your biofield—which is comprised of both measurable electromagnetic energy and so-called subtle energy. While the electricity in the body is widely accepted as fact, Western science does not agree that you have this energy field around you, despite the law of physics that states everything with an electric current running through it has a magnetic field around it. Our current paradigm of biology and medicine is still firmly entrenched in a mechanical worldview that treats concepts like life energy, energy medicine, biofields, and the like as myth, despite mounting evidence to the contrary. But that is beginning to change. The work of a small and earnest group of researchers has shown not only that this field exists but also that it may provide the blueprint for order and coherence that underlies our physiologies.

My view, founded on my own clinical experience and increasingly supported by reputable science, is that the biofield and the subtle (or punitive, meaning, "rumored to exist") energy of which it is in part comprised is not something separate from the electricity that our hearts and brains run on. We've created a wall between the two in our minds, no doubt stemming from the challenge of defining and measuring subtle energy. However, these different forms of energy, rather than being distinct entities, exist as more of a spectrum or gradient. Along this spectrum, subtle energy appears to be simply a higher harmonic of the denser, measurable electromagnetic energy that's present throughout our biological systems. It's the same thing, only weaker and following slightly different laws—think water and water vapor.

While Western science has yet to quantify the subtle energy that makes up the biofield, other cultures, especially ancient Indian or Vedic cultures, describe it extensively. Another word for this energy is *bioplasma:* a diffuse, weakly charged magnetic fluid that surrounds all living beings. Like any fluid, it can be of varying viscosities and densities. In Biofield Tuning, we view the human biofield as a bioplasmic toroid-shaped bubble that surrounds the body at a distance of about five to six feet on the sides and two to three feet at the top and bottom. This magnetic bubble is bounded at its outer edge by a protective double-layer plasma membrane that is much like the earth's ionosphere and the sun's heliosphere.

While the picture I'm describing is fairly different from what we've been taught about our bodies, it's really not such a foreign concept. The electrical nature of our bodies is something that's been hidden in plain view. We recognize the pieces—we know that there is some electrical activity going on in our brains and our hearts—and yet the full picture of our electromagnetic nature hasn't really been put together in most people's minds.

That's understandable considering the way we've been encultured to think of ourselves as chemical-mechanical beings. The standard-model perspective (known in science as the *mechanist* view) suggests that any electrical activity in the body is a result of physiological activity, while on the other side of the aisle, the *vitalists* take the opposite view, arguing that electromagnetic and subtle energy activity is what *gives rise to our physiology*. According to the vitalists, the body is not only composed of physical, mechanical, and chemical components but also of a resonating electromagnetism, with each cell, organ, and system contributing to a symphony of complex standing waves of many different frequencies.

Looking at life and the body from a mechanist perspective provides the basis for Western medicine, while looking at things from a vitalist perspective offers a scientific foundation for many types of complementary and alternative medicine, including modalities like Biofield Tuning, Reiki, homeopathy, music therapy, and shamanic healing. With the new research that's emerging, we are moving toward a more holistic understanding that encompasses both of these perspectives: wave and particle, vitalist and mechanist, scientific evidence and spiritual awareness.

DISCOVERING THE BIOFIELD IN SCIENCE

Dating back to the eighteenth century, a number of intrepid researchers have conducted pioneering (but largely ignored) research into our electromagnetic nature. While there were and are a great many physicians and scientists who have explored health and life from this angle, here are just a few of them.

In 1773, German physician Franz Anton Mesmer began using magnets for healing and claimed that he detected a magnetic field surrounding the body. Mesmer proposed that everything in the universe, including the human body, was governed by a magnetic fluid that could become imbalanced, causing illness. Based on his study of "animal magnetism," as he called it, Mesmer formulated a theory of energy flow in the body that roughly aligns with that of Chinese medicine. Through his clinical work and experiments, he came to view health as the free circulation of life force through the body's many energy channels and illness as the result of blockages in this flow.

I was astonished to find in Mesmer's work a protocol that so elegantly mirrored my own. In a process not unlike Biofield Tuning, Mesmer actually used metal rods (and later, his hands) to shift the flow of the body's magnetic fluid. And he was also using sound! He used a contraption, invented by Benjamin Franklin, that had round glasses on a spindle in a tray of water that he would spin to create a sound similar to a singing bowl and then work with his hands on the field of his patient while the tone was sounding. Two hundred fifty years ago, Mesmer was doing almost exactly what I've been doing since the '90s!

The theory behind Mesmer's protocol also echoed the hypotheses that I had been forming based on my observations. He suggested that dislodging energy blockages in the magnetic field around the body could create an initial healing crisis or detox reaction, followed by restored flow and improved health. Mesmer, like me, observed that these blockages in the energy field were correlated with blockages within the body. Where energy does not flow, pathologies would inevitably arise. (Anyone familiar with Chinese medicine will see the parallel here on the importance of chi flowing properly through the system.) Where my work seemed to take things a step further was to show that the coherent tones produced by an activated tuning fork apparently act as a conductor of magnetism in that they have the capacity to unblock the flow of life force or free up "frozen" bioplasma.

Mesmer was ahead of his time. His "magnetic fluid" was derided as pseudoscience, and he was condemned for his work and was barred from practicing medicine. Part of this dismissal of fields from the establishment comes from the division of science and religion that has characterized our investigations of the natural world for over three centuries. Things having to do with "soul" and "spirit" were removed from hard science and put in the domain of religion. I have come to see what we call the *biofield* as the same thing that we call *soul*—and as far as science is concerned, you don't have a soul! All you have to do is consider a powerful soul singer singing in a fiery way from her electric body and you can easily see the correlation.

In the mid–twentieth century, Yale anatomy professor Harold Saxton Burr became one of the first Americans to do extensive research on the electromagnetic fields surrounding matter. From 1937 until the 1970s, he conducted many experiments on these energy fields, which he dubbed *L-fields*. These electrodynamic fields, which he claimed to be present in all living things, became the subject of his 1973 book *The Fields of Life*. Burr believed that L-fields were the blueprints of living matter. If a disturbed energy field could be detected and corrected, he suggested, pathology in the organism could be prevented from arising. Burr's work also wasn't accepted in his time, likely due to its challenge to the chemical model upon which the modern pharmacopoeia was being built. While his research was largely pushed aside, it became the basis for the seminal work of American orthopedic surgeon and electrophysiology researcher Robert O. Becker, author of the classic 1985 book *The Body Electric: Electromagnetism and the Foundation of Life.*

Becker, often referred to as the father of electromedicine, conducted fifty years' worth of research on human bioelectricity. He discovered, among other things, that animals show a direct current of electric charge, which is measurable from their body surfaces. One of Becker's big accomplishments was helping to bring credibility to the practice of acupuncture in the eyes of Western medicine, which he did by proving acupuncture points to be regions of higher electrical conductivity than the tissue surrounding them. (It's worth noting that Becker had also become concerned about how non-natural electromagnetic fields might be affecting human health, a line of research he never had the opportunity to pursue.)

Like Burr, Becker described the electromagnetic fields in and around the body as the sort of primary causal force, or blueprint, for the organization of the physical body—a notion later reflected in British biologist Rupert Sheldrake's concepts of morphic resonance and morphogenetic fields. Sheldrake suggested that we are informed by fields of information that are both causal and generative and that we are constantly adding to those fields as we accumulate life experiences. It's like we're carrying around our own personal cloud storage systems or Akashic records that carry our entire histories, as well as all the encoded information that informs our physical bodies.

The conventional thinking is that our electromagnetic fields can only be detected a few millimeters off the body. But our understanding of subtle energy has been limited by our ability to detect it. We can't use a voltmeter to measure subtle signals any more than we can use a measuring cup to measure water vapor. However, many people are surprised to hear of a device that was invented back in 1964 called the SQUID, or superconducting quantum interference device—an extremely sensitive magnetometer, capable of measuring the biomagnetic field produced by a single heartbeat, muscle twitch, or pattern of neural activity in the brain. The SQUID magnetometer has been able to detect a faint magnetic field as far as twelve feet away from the body.

Using SQUID and other devices, there have more recently been some notable scientific efforts to measure the subtle energy of the biofield. Dr. William Tiller at Stanford developed a subtle energy detector with which they were able to demonstrate the existence of an energy field that is not in the known electromagnetic spectrum, and to show that this energy responds to human intention and focus. Dr. Valerie Hunt at UCLA also developed a high-frequency instrument that records the bioelectrical energy that emanates from the body's surface—which she hypothesized to oscillate at significantly higher frequencies than EKGs or EEGs can measure. Hunt's work proved that energy radiating from the body's surface gives off frequencies one thousand times faster than any other known electrical activity of the body.

Hunt conducted research using an electromagnetically shielded, or mu-metal, room and found that when electromagnetism was removed from the room, people "went to pieces," having emotional breakdowns for no discernable reasons. When ambient electromagnetic energy was restored to the room, participants found themselves feeling fine again. This seems to imply that the presence of EM fields is necessary for the organism to maintain a sense of coherence and "togetherness"—adding weight to the blueprint hypothesis of myself and scientists like Becker, Sheldrake, and Burr.

In the early 2000s, biofield science began to take off with the seminal work of UCLA biophysicist Beverly Rubik. In her 2002 paper "The Biofield Hypothesis: Its Biophysical Basis and Role in Medicine," Rubik describes the biofield as a complex, weak electromagnetic field that utilizes electromagnetic "bioinformation" for self-regulation. The field, as she presents it, is a light grid of near-instantaneous communication that underlies the much slower chemical processes that it gives rise to—challenging the mechanist view that chemical reactions are what give rise to human bioelectricity. Rubik also makes the case that this field is what accounts for some of the rapid and wide-ranging effects of certain alternative and complementary medicine therapies that claim to work on an energetic level.

Rubik's biofield hypothesis begins to provide a scientific foundation for how, and why, healing modalities like Reiki, Biofield Tuning, Pranic Healing, and Therapeutic Touch work. This is very significant. What we call *energy medicine* has been controversial and cast aside, largely because a theory for how and why these therapies work has yet to be fully developed, nor does there seem to want to be one.

The work of Rubik and other biofield scientists showed that by interacting with the organism's biofield, these modalities seem to exert an effect on homeodynamics—the organizing intelligence of the body that is always seeking to promote healing and maintain order and balance. Research in the years since has continued to demonstrate the efficacy of healing approaches that target the body's energy system. A systematic review of sixty-six clinical trials, conducted in 2010, showed that biofield therapies demonstrate strong and significant effects in reducing pain and anxiety, and other palliative effects.[1]

In April 2020, my friend and colleague Dr. Shamini Jain and her partners at the Consciousness and Healing Initiative (CHI) released a comprehensive report titled "Subtle Energy & Biofield Healing: Evidence, Practice, & Future Directions." This effort assembled a library of roughly 6,200 publications in subtle energy and biofield healing, as well as a thoroughly reviewed and mapped subset of 396 clinical studies of subtle energy and biofield healing modalities for various health conditions. This wealth of information is available for free at www.chi.is.

---

1. S. Jain and P. Mills, "Biofield Therapies: Helpful or Full of Hype? A Best Evidence Synthesis," *International Journal of Behavioral Medicine* 17 no. 1 (2010): 1–16.

THE STRUCTURE OF THE BIOFIELD

Modern biofield science has yet to detail the structure and activity of the body's energy field. But if we look back to ancient Vedic and Chinese medicine systems, we find a codification of the workings of a life force energy in the body that kept us alive and healthy, and when blocked, created illness and low vitality. They understood everything in life as energy, electricity, vibration; and they knew that in the body, this energy—which was constantly in motion, flowing, and circulating—had to be kept in balance and harmony. In fact, the word *chi* translates into "electricity," but the concept of chi embraces the subtler aspects of electricity that our conventional understanding does not quite go so far as to define.

This life force energy was known to flow through certain channels, known as *nadis* in the yogic tradition and *meridians* in Chinese medicine. The ancient yogic texts, the Upanishads, describe the nadis as a near-infinite network of tubular organs or channels of energy flow felt throughout the body, with the seven chakras being the epicenters and origins of this energy flow. From the chakras, which are like transponders of particular frequencies, the energy then moves outward throughout and beyond the body through the pathways of the nadis, becoming finer and more diffuse the farther away it travels from these main energy centers.

Of all the seventy-two thousand nadis, the three most important are the Ida, Pingala, and Sushumna. The Sushumna is our central channel, the electromagnetically neutral axis that travels vertically up and down the spine at the midline of the body. The negatively charged Ida, which starts to the left of the base of the spine, and the positively charged Pingala, to the right of the spine, twirl around each other along the Sushumna, representing the masculine and feminine energies. Interestingly, the twirling Ida and Pingala mirror the shape of Birkeland currents, the geomagnetic field lines connecting the earth's magnetosphere to the earth's high-altitude ionosphere—and both of these twisting currents mirror the double helix shape of DNA. As above, so below!

The biofield, on many different levels, presents a fractal rendering of what we see in the earth and in interstellar space. Birkeland currents, the long, spiraling ropes of electricity that connect interstellar objects, are made up of a positive and negative charge, demonstrating what's called *long-range attraction* and *short-range repulsion*. When they come into this tension between the forces of attraction and repulsion, these currents spin and spiral bidirectionally. This spiral motion of opposing forces is a sacred geometric design that can be seen throughout the natural world.

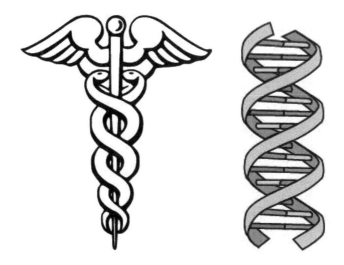

All electromagnetic energy comes in polarities of positive and negative, due to the fact that electricity stems from the phenomenon of positive and negative charge. Polarity is a fundamental property of not only electromagnetism but all matter. In Chinese medicine, they describe these two fundamental and opposing energies in the body and in all nature as yin and yang, representing the masculine (positive) and feminine (negative) energies.

The bioplasmic field around the body, which appears to be composed at the atomic level of free electrons, ions, and protons, also demonstrates this balance of positive and negative particles. These charged energies spin around each other in what's known as a *torsion force*—a kind of twisting, spiraling motion. Torsion waves travel in either a right-hand or a left-hand direction, and depending on the direction of the spin, the energy takes on either a positive or negative polarity. Everything in nature is moved by this fundamental spiraling motion—the way water flows, the way blood spirals through our veins, the way energy flows within the toroidal field of the human body. These torsion waves spin within the toroidal, or doughnut-shaped, biofield. Anything that is electromagnetic is going to have this toroidal field around it.

As we've seen, the toroid is another pattern that repeats itself in nature. The earth has an atmosphere that's bounded by a magnetic layer—the inner layer is called the *ionosphere* and the outer layer is called the *magnetosphere*—which is an area of greater electrical charge that bounds our atmosphere. We all learned in elementary school science that this creates a boundary of sorts so that things like radio waves and the Schumann resonance bounce off it and create standing waves in the atmosphere. The sun also has its heliosphere, which defines the outer edge of the solar system.

The human biofield is a fractal rendering of the same idea. I see the outer layer of the biofield as a double-layer membrane, and I perceive it to be about an inch and a half thick. Just as we have these standing waves within the earth's atmosphere, we have standing waves within our own fields. I talked in chapter 1 about how these standing waves seem to be magnetically encoded with our memories, and they move away from us as we generate them (hence the rings-on-a-tree analogy).

This outer boundary comes together above the head and below the feet to form a channel spiraling down the middle—this is the central channel, the Sushumna. In Biofield Tuning, we begin every session by activating what we call the Earth Star and Sun Star energy centers. These points are the positive and negative terminals of the body's battery. These are points at either end of the central channel of the toroid, the spiraling pathway of energy that goes down the core of the body. The Earth Star brings up what we call the *ascending current*, the negative charge from the surface of the earth, and the Sun Star brings down the positive or *descending* current from the sun and stars. To get the electric body primed and amplified, we amplify the main current that travels along the center of your being. I think of it as activating your inner lightning rod. Being anchored in the central channel is what it means, electromagnetically, to be *centered* in your own being.

THE BIOPHOTON HYPOTHESIS

In my attempt to decipher the nature of the "stuff" I was finding in people's energy fields, I wasn't finding any precedent in Western science, nor was I getting much insight from the yogic system, Chinese medicine, or any other ancient healing tradition. While what I was working with could easily be called *chi,* I was trying to find words and concepts in the Western model to describe the phenomena I was encountering. But as I went deeper into emerging research on the biofield, a hypothesis began brewing in my mind.

When I became aware that the perturbations I was finding in the field were related to stress and trauma and that there was energy trapped in these places, I began to consider that it was *biophotons* that I was dealing with. Biophotons are particles of light in the ultraviolet and low visible light range that are produced by biological systems. Biophotons were first discovered in 1923 by Russian scientist Alexander Gurwitsch, who also originated the morphogenetic field theory that Rupert Sheldrake has popularized.

More recently studied and described by German biophysicist Fritz-Albert Popp in the 1970s, biophotons serve the key functions of cell-to-cell communications, stimulation of biochemical reactions, and coordination within the body. Biophotons, in essence, are quanta of coherent light that are emitted and absorbed by the DNA in our cells—meaning that our cells are literally radiating with light! The DNA of every cell creates light, and that light is a highly structured electromagnetic wave that the cell uses to communicate with other cells. Interestingly, Popp found that the spiral structure of DNA is an ideal arrangement for storing and emitting light through its rhythmic contractions.

Their main purpose of biophotons seems to be communication. To-gether, they appear to create a coherent electromagnetic field throughout the body that uses electromagnetic frequencies for near-instantaneous (speed-of-light) communication throughout the system—and they appear to play an important role in the maintenance of order and coherence.

Biophotons are present not only in the body but also in its surrounding biofield. According to biophysicist Dietrich Klinghardt, who is doing fascinating work in this area, this light that exists just beyond our physical bodies fulfills an important biological purpose, too. As he puts it, some of the light waves that radiate out from our cells leave the body and create a highly structured light field around us, which he calls a *coherent field*. His description of the coherent field, which perfectly echoes my own understanding of the biofield, is that it carries the information of all the body's cells and the memory of every event that the organism has been exposed to. That field carries the information of every cell in the body, and it engages in a bidirectional information transfer with people, plants, animals, and energies in our environment. The field sends back information it takes in from outside to the cells in the body. This is also a helpful framework for understanding how our lives become a reflection of our energy fields. If there are a lot of chaotic waveforms in your field, you're going to be bringing that information into your interactions and likely attracting the same kind of waveforms.

How much light do our bodies emit? There appears to be a sweet spot of ideal biophoton emissions: not too little, not too much. Popp's work showed that healthy organisms emit a certain amount of *coherent* light, and that dysfunctional cells emit a low amplitude of chaotic, or noncoherent, light—in other words, the chaotic waveforms that I was finding in the field!

Stress or illness seems to cause an excessive leaking of noncoherent light into the field. Research using biophoton imaging devices has shown that when an organism is under stress, it emits more biophotons—a leaking of life force that seems to result in a loss of order and integrity throughout the system. We literally leak out light as a result of stress and trauma. We lose our sparkle. This is a real scientific description of how the light in our eyes and the brightness in our beings go dim as a result of stress and trauma. Experiments have been conducted that use biophoton counters and cameras to compare biophoton activity in different subjects, like monks in meditation versus individuals under stress. While the meditating monks give off very little light, people under stress are emitting large amounts of light out of their bodies and into the field around them. You can bet that if you looked at the photonic emissions of a person who was just in a car accident or recently lost someone they love, they're going to be shedding a huge amount of light.

I actually was able to conduct an experiment using Biofield Tuning and a biophoton counter while working on my Ph.D. at the California Institute for Human Science. I hypothesized that a tune-up would decrease biophotonic output from a classmate's throat chakra. We did a measurement first, I conducted the session, and then we took another reading. The photonic emissions from this part of her body dropped 22 percent, supporting the notion that it is healthier for the body to be in a state of energy conservation and not leaking light and life force.

My current theory is that what I'm finding with my tuning fork in these areas of distortion and resistance are incoherent waveforms trapping the photons/energy/light from flowing freely through the systems (and likely also what are called *biophonons*, the lower-frequency, sound equivalent of biophotons) that we've leaked during periods of our lives when we were under stress. Rather than being lost and gone forever, the light and energy we lost during those turbulent times appears to stay in our own atmosphere, and we can actually return it to its rightful place in the body. It's almost like reversing the aging process. I've come to understand aging as just the *loss of light over time.* As we go through life and take hits, we lose energy and information and order. But we can slow, and even reverse, the aging process by cultivating photonic density. I can say with some certainty that this is possible, because I look and feel younger at fifty-one than I did at thirty-five and didn't yet have the resources I do now for managing my stress levels. If you could see into a child's energy field, you would notice that they are very photonically dense. Their photons are densely packed. That's youth, vigor, energy! Adults who have been through the wringer become photonically diffuse as their energy ends up scattered throughout their field.

When I comb energy through the field and deposit it back into the body, I have the sense of literally returning the person's light to them.

When clients finish a session, the response is universally the same: "I feel lighter." People look and feel lighter. With an understanding of the bio-photonic nature of our bodies, this response makes quite a lot of sense!

Biophoton research is a growing field of study that's yielding some exciting outcomes. It was only around ten years ago that research on bio-photon emissions started appearing in American scientific journals, and since then, fascinating discoveries have been made—like the finding that individual neurons in the brain give off light and that biophotons in the brain seem to play a key role in neural information transfer. Our brain cells are actually communicating through light! If you've ever looked at a map of neurons in the brain, it looks strikingly like the webs of light connecting stars and galaxies across the cosmos. (The number of neurons in the brain is roughly the same as the number of galaxies in the observable universe!) Further research on biophotons in the brain may help us to better understand different states of consciousness and higher-order brain functions like perception, emotions, and creativity, according to Klinghardt.

Another fascinating study, published in the journal *Neuroscience Letters*, found that when people imagine light in the dark, they actually show increased biophoton emissions from the head—suggesting that the halos painted around saints in religious art may be an indication of elevated, illuminated thinking!

This new physiology of light may prove invaluable in bridging science and spirituality. It's actual proof that we are light beings! When the ancient Tibetan yogis talked about the "rainbow body" that is illuminated from within, they were accurately describing our biology. As Carl Sagan said, "We are the stuff of the stars."

CELLS: YOUR ELECTRICAL SUPERCONDUCTORS

To really understand our light bodies, we have to travel down to the cellular level.

We were all taught in school to look at cell biology in terms of chemistry. We learn about this lock-and-key mechanism whereby molecules are bumping around and getting in and out of the cell. But what we weren't taught is the electromagnetic function of our cells and the way they communicate through light.

Cells are the building blocks of human bioelectricity. They generate tiny electric currents as a result of charge flow and changes in membrane potential and thus generate tiny magnetic fields. These currents are created by the flow of electrically charged particles like calcium, potassium, sodium, or magnesium (also known as ions) that flow in and out of your cell membranes. The flow of these positively and negatively charged particles across the cell membrane is what generates the electrical currents that power our bodies. In turn, our cells are supported by the continual flow of electrons being delivered by oxygen and food.

The electrical signaling function of our cells is imperative to our overall health. Disease is both the cause and the result of disruptions in this signaling system. It's been discovered in recent years that cancer cells steal electricity from healthy cells. Research published last year in the journal *Nature* showed that certain types of deadly brain tumors known as *gliomas* work their way into the brain's electrical network and hijack the signal of healthy nerve cells, which they use to fuel their own growth. One of the study's authors, Heidelberg University neuroscientist Dr. Frank Winkler, described their behavior as "vampire"-like.

We now know that our cells emit sound as well as light. Not only do your cells radiate light, they also make music! In a 2018 article published in the journal of the British Society for Gene and Cell Therapy, Dr. Liam Hurst wrote that the human body is home to "ten trillion tiny musical maestros." This cellular symphony was discovered in 2001 when UCLA biophysicist Jim Gimzewski's work revealed that the vibrations emitted by certain cells as they divide and multiply can be amplified into audible sound. What do cells sound like? "Beautiful," Gimzewski said.

But when Gimzewski and his team dropped the cells into ethanol, they began to release a piercing screech as they died. The researchers also discovered that things like environmental changes and genetic mutations could change the pitch, frequency, and volume of a cell's song. Other studies showed that cancerous cells produce a sound that is completely unlike that of healthy cells. One researcher described the sound of a group of cancer cells as "horribly out-of-tune." With further research, the study of cell sounds, *sonocytology,* could offer tremendous insight into health and disease on a cellular level—even allowing doctors to "hear" disease in its early stages.

"This biological warning siren may allow the sound of an unhealthy cell to become a standard diagnostic tool—catching disease far earlier than a battery of current diagnostic tests ever could," Hurst wrote.

This research is an exciting validation of the potential of what we're doing in Biofield Tuning: listening to the song of our cells and tuning out-of-tune cells so as to return the body to a natural state of harmony and coherence.

MICROTUBULES: CONSCIOUSNESS ON A CELLULAR LEVEL

Here's yet another fascinating function of your cells: On the surface of every cell membrane are cilia, which are like little antennas. These cilia house microtubules, which vibrate in response to incoming vibrational information from our environment. My hypothesis is that these are actually the antennas that are receiving and transmitting the information that's held in the field so that the cell is informing the field and the field is informing the cell. Microtubules may be an actual biological apparatus for sensing "vibes" through the magnetic medium of the field. I call it our *wave sense.* It's not some kind of vague intuition that some women have. It's how our bodies are built. These antennas are constantly receiving and transmitting the information of the cell. This explains a lot of how the tuning forks work in the field: When you get into the frequency range for the signal of a cell and that cell has a lot of dissonance in it, the dissonance is what's being transmitted and picked up by the fork. Then the coherent vibration that the fork is introducing gets received, and it sends that information of order and harmony back to the cell.

In his classic 2005 book *The Biology of Belief,* Dr. Bruce Lipton explains the key function of these antennas:

Receptor antennas can also read vibrational energy fields such as light,
sound, and radio frequencies. The antennas on the energy receptors
vibrate like tuning forks. If an energy vibration in the environment
resonates with a receptor's antenna, it will alter the protein's charge,
causing the receptor to change shape. Because these receptors can read
energy fields, the notion that only physical molecules can impact cell
physiology is outmoded.

The academic community is currently exploring whether microtubules could potentially play a role in consciousness. One theory from Oxford mathematical physicist Sir Roger Penrose, not yet widely accepted, suggests that it is the quantum vibrations of microtubules in neurons that gives rise to brain wave rhythms—and that treating microtubule vibrations could benefit neurological and cognitive health conditions.

"The origin of consciousness reflects our place in the universe, the nature of our existence. Did consciousness evolve from complex computations among brain neurons, as most scientists assert? Or has consciousness, in some sense, been here all along, as spiritual approaches maintain?" ask Penrose and his colleague Stuart Hameroff in a 2014 review of the theory. "This opens a potential Pandora's Box, but our theory accommodates both these views, suggesting consciousness derives from quantum vibrations in microtubules, protein polymers inside brain neurons, which both govern neuronal and synaptic function, and connect brain processes to self-organizing processes in the fine scale, 'proto-conscious' quantum structure of reality."

Since the theory was first developed in the mid-'90s, some promising new research on Alzheimer's patients has lent support. Scientists have recently discovered that microtubules start to fail in the brains of patients with Alzheimer's. Based on my own understanding, if our memories are indeed stored in standing waves in the field, and if the microtubule is an apparatus for retrieving those memories but the microtubule is not functioning properly, then it would make sense that these people are not able to retrieve their memories. The memories are not physically located in the brain; they're actually stored in the field (or perhaps they are stored in both). I once did a group session on improving memory and brain health, and I worked specifically on the microtubules in the brain. When I focused on the microtubules, I was amazed by just how much information they held. What I discovered was that some of them are actually crouched and pulling in. It's possible that this is a pattern that dates back to a dissociative response to childhood trauma. If you think about growing up in a home where you had to protect yourself or draw your energy in, all these little antennas for sensing are not going to be happy and alert and paying close attention to the environment. They're going to have suffered just like you did and respond with that patterning of pulling inward.

As we'll now explore, it is our emotions—the electromagnetic waves of feeling that constantly flow through our being—that determine, more than any other single factor, the state of our physical, biochemical, and electric health.

6

Your Electromagnetic Emotions

Several years ago, researchers at MIT's Computer Science and Artificial Intelligence Laboratory created a device that uses radio waves to detect human emotion. The shoebox-size emotion recognition device, called EQ Radio, works by bouncing wireless signals off a person and analyzing the signal that comes back—which is influenced by things like breathing, heart rate, and minute vibrations on the surface of the skin caused by the pumping of blood. The radio waves are impacted by these vibrations, and the returning signals are then analyzed by a computer to detect changes in a person's emotional state.

When I first learned of this, I was amazed by how similar this was to what I have been doing (albeit in a slightly more primitive fashion!) with my tuning forks. I am able to detect a person's emotions (either a current emotion, a past emotion that is stuck somewhere in the field, or an underlying emotional baseline) by using the forks to bounce a signal off the person and listening to the vibration that comes back—similar to the way a bat or dolphin navigates using echolocation. Both of these techniques are able to recognize human emotions through the analysis of vibrations, or waves, in the person's energy field.

Our emotions are not just chemical and mechanical. An emotion is a waveform. It is a fundamentally electromagnetic phenomenon that gives rise to chemical and physiological changes like heart rate increase or decrease, muscle tension, and breathing rhythm—but the vibrational aspect is primary. If we look at the etymology of the word *emotion,* it reveals that an emotion is a moving thing, it's "in motion." The word itself is derived from the French *émouvoir,* which means "to stir up." This tells us that an emotion is a thing that's stirred up and moves around inside us when life plays our heartstrings.

As a waveform, an emotion naturally rises up, crests in our awareness, and then falls away. This is both an electrical and a chemical phenomenon. As that wave rises up, chemicals are generated. The work of Candace Pert, a neuroscientist and pharmacologist formerly with the National Institutes of Health and who is credited with discovering the brain's opiate receptors, showed that there is actually a chemical, molecular component to emotion. When we feel something, a set of electrical impulses as well as a molecule of emotion is generated. Different emotions, of course, have different chemical compositions. Fear creates adrenaline, for instance, while love creates oxytocin, and excitement creates dopamine. The brain and gut generate molecules that carry the vibration of that particular wave, and the waveform carries them throughout the body. Those molecules go into circulation, and we feel the vibration of that waveform.

One way to think about it is that our emotions are magnetic and our thoughts are electric. Magnetic fields guide electric currents: Our feelings are primary, and our thoughts follow. When we work with our emotions, we're shifting the magnetic field, which is then shifting the way the electric current is running through the body—and ultimately showing up in certain mental and physical patterns. Physical pain is often the final manifestation of an emotional pattern in the magnetic field. If I have a pain in my right shoulder, I have too much electric current running through those wires. The Biofield Tuning approach is to find where the magnetic field is stuck there and shift the magnetic field so that the electric current will flow differently through the body. Wherever there is stuck energy in the field, there is corresponding tension in the body. When we release the resistance in the magnetic field, the electric resistance and corresponding tension in the body also lets go.

Let's dig a little deeper here. Magnetism is traditionally associated with the feminine, yin principle and electricity with the masculine, yang principle. The feminine element is emotion; it's music and sound and feeling. The masculine element is thought; it's electricity and light. The magnetic field is diffuse and all-encompassing, while the electricity is more of the focused charge. As the feminine has been oppressed by the masculine in modern patriarchal cultures, intellect, reason, and logic have been favored over emotion and intuition, which also plays out in the way that we've repressed our feeling sense and overengaged our thinking apparatus.

We've even cut this awareness of the magnetic field out of our understanding of life! Our collective consciousness is mirrored in nature. Scientists have found that the earth's magnetic field is decreasing. Over the last four or five thousand years, according to geological history, the magnetic field has been in decline. And any time a magnetic field is decreasing, the electric current is increasing.

This is what we've seen in our society. The patriarchy has risen; the development of thought, mind, intellect, science, and technology—the electric charge—has increased. The elimination of the feminine—the element of nourishment, caring, emotion, and wholeness—has occurred in so many different places in our culture, and it's also happened to the earth. Is the magnetic field declining because of the way that human consciousness has been changing, or vice versa? What's the cause, and what's the effect? It's impossible to say. Either way, we have seen the decline of the feminine principle along with the decline of our collective emotional health and our understanding of magnetism at the same time.

The weakening of the magnetosphere offers an interesting perspective on the way we're seeing things falling apart in the world right now. Remember the mu-room study? When people were placed in a room where the magnetic field was removed, they went to pieces. What we're seeing in the world today is that we don't have this magnetic insulation, so nerves are fraying, the electric current is amping up, and everything is becoming very electric and intense. When we're not contained by the magnetosphere, we're not being held by the Mother.

If we want to change our minds and bodies, we need to start with our emotions. So much of New Age thought, including the work of some brilliant minds like Joe Dispenza, focuses on the notion of "change your thinking, change your life." There's truth to this, but at the same time, changing our thinking doesn't work so well if we're not also addressing the underlying feelings that are guiding the thoughts.

We really need to change *the way we feel,* and the only way to change the way we feel is by getting in touch with whatever undigested emotions are hanging out in our biofields. And there are a lot of them in most people! If you've got all this guilt or shame or anger that you're not owning—or that you're suppressing with wine or sugar or overworking—then those unexpressed emotions are going to undermine you. They're going to cause self-sabotage. They're going to get in the way of you changing your thinking and changing your life.

You can think *I am rich and abundant* all you want, but if you don't feel abundant because you have a bunch of stories of lack and "not enough" created by a backlog of shame that you've never addressed, then you're not going to get very far. You need to have all your vibrations in phase with each other in inner alignment and inner unity, and then you become more powerful. You become more magnetic. You start to attract whatever you want, because 100 percent of you is on board. You're vibrating that feeling of abundance in your field, and what you vibrate is what you experience.

It is my observation that virtually all undisciplined thinking and inability to control our minds and behaviors come from the ants in our pants caused by unresolved emotions. You can try to shift your electric thinking all you want, but if your magnetic field is stuck in some emotion that never got expressed, you're going to keep sabotaging yourself, because that emotion is going to keep seeking to find its expression. It's going to keep trying to fulfill its destiny as a waveform, which is expression. And it will keep undermining your thinking and your behavior until that emotion reaches its destiny of expression.

To one degree or another, we all have a vibrational backlog of unprocessed emotions. These old emotions become signal jammers that put us in a state of incoherence and create a feeling of "stuckness." Most people come to see me because they are stuck in some kind of pattern that's creating unhealthy consequences in their bodies and their lives. There is a good reason why we say in Biofield Tuning, "Better out than in!"

The heart of what I teach is effective emotional management: learning to dance with our emotions. When we learn to accept our emotions as a healthy and natural part of life, we enter into a fluid relationship with them, whereby we simply allow whatever emotion is arising at the moment to arise and do its thing. We let it out in some way, and then we move on.

Unexpressed emotions generate stress, and ultimately, the state of our health comes down to how we manage stress. Even the Centers for Disease Control and Prevention says that 85 percent of chronic illness is stress-related. Stress is emotion, plain and simple. Our emotional response to a situation, rather than the situation itself, is what causes most stress. The solution in our current health care model is to give people drugs, but what we really need is to identify what's going on below the level of our symptoms. What's going on with almost every single person I've worked with is that there are unexpressed and undigested emotions in their bodies that they don't know what to do with.

THE SECRET LIFE OF BURIED EMOTIONS

As a waveform, an emotion rises up into our awareness so that we can recognize it, express it, acknowledge the message it carries, and use that information to guide our decisions about how we will respond to a particular situation.

Emotions naturally ebb and flow like the tide—if we allow them to. More often, we do whatever we can to stop an oncoming wave in its tracks. There are countless ways to arrest the movement of a waveform: taking a pill, eating a chocolate bar, pouring a glass of wine, going shopping, sitting in front of a screen, or just overriding it with a noisy inner monologue. Capitalism provides us with limitless opportunities to avoid our emotions.

If an emotion is generated and then it is suppressed with alcohol or sugar or anything else, that emotion does not go away. When a wave's motion is arrested, the molecules that were generated don't get digested or recycled. They stay in our system, and they have to find a home. Guilt might settle in your hips and thighs, while anger is most likely to go hang out in your liver. Sadness may find some corner of your heart or lungs to claim for itself. Our systems end up becoming full of these molecules of waveforms that are just waiting to break.

There is a saying in the therapy world: "Emotions buried alive never die." This has certainly been my observation while working in the field. Just about everything that I pick up with my tuning forks as resistance carries some kind of emotional charge, whether it's anger, sadness, guilt, regret, fear, or some complex combination of many emotions melded together. If we do not express and release these emotions as they are arising, then we will be forced to carry them around with us—for years, decades, and maybe even lifetimes. By using my tuning forks to locate, unearth, and release the trapped emotions that have become frozen in the field and the body, what I'm essentially doing is helping that emotion to fulfill its destiny.

Disease is often the body's last resort to making the emotion heard. Even the medical establishment is beginning to acknowledge the link between emotional suppression and disease—particularly in the case of autoimmune diseases. Mounting evidence has shown that unprocessed emotions, often stemming from childhood trauma, may play a significant role in autoimmunity. The respected Canadian physician Dr. Gabor Maté wrote in his 2003 book, *When The Body Says No: Exploring the Stress-Disease Connection,* that "underlying emotional repression was an ever-present factor" in nearly every autoimmune patient he has worked with.

On a chemical level, when we suppress the emotion before it crests, it has to go find a little hidey-hole in the body to hang out in. It'll go knock on a cell's door and say, "Can I come in here and hide? Because nobody wants to deal with me right now." When we experience chronic, low-level sadness or anger or anxiety, it's because you have all those molecules just hanging out in your cells. Over time, those chemicals hiding out in a certain organ or part of the body disrupt the blueprint, and disease or disorder is the result.

When we unearth an emotion and iron it out in the field, all of a sudden, the cells are going back into their blueprint and saying, "Oh, this little molecule of sadness—you're not in the blueprint anymore. You're getting kicked to the curb." You take it out into the body, and it goes into circulation to fulfill its destiny. Emotions and physical detox reactions can arise as those chemicals are released from the system, which can be uncomfortable but generally pass fairly quickly.

I have done a lot of suppressing sadness in my lifetime—what turned out to be generations of it. It was an emotional process to work through that backlog. But once I did, I just felt lighter and brighter. Those background feelings just fade away. It takes a little time, but if you keep at this work, you systematically get all those old emotions out of your field and out of your cells. The old stories and patterns and rhythms depattern, and then something new takes their place: gratitude, joy, playfulness, creativity, spontaneity.

The goal is not to get rid of all these emotions so that we are no longer emotional. You're still going to be emotional. Even after years of clearing out my emotional baggage, I nevertheless cry very easily. If something goes through my newsfeed that's either really beautiful or really sad, I'm going to sit there and cry, but then I'll snap back into neutral. But because of this natural flow of emotions, I also laugh easily, play easily, and feel gratitude easily. The goal, as I see it, is to get rid of the backlog so that when you do feel an emotion, it's not lighting up every other backlogged emotion that's in your body. You're not having a disproportionate emotional reaction because of all the undigested, unexpressed sentiments that you're dragging along behind you. This is about getting rid of baggage, traveling light. Whatever emotions arise will be much more manageable once you've dredged up the backlog and gotten it out of the body.

There's no shame in having an emotional backlog to address (welcome to the human experience!). Whether it's fear, sadness, rage, hate, shame, or jealousy, we all suppress emotions to some degree or other—some of us quite valiantly! But our emotions will continue to try to get our attention, like anything buried alive might. If we don't recognize them for what they are and find healthy ways to express them, they will find their own way to express themselves—in sickness or disease, tumultuous life situations, or a mental or emotional breakdown.

The bottom line is that as humans, we all experience the full spectrum of emotions, whether we recognize them or not. If we do not express our emotions in a conscious and healthy manner, they will be expressed subconsciously in our bodies and in our lives.

PURPLE-WASHING AND SPIRITUAL BYPASSING

I coined the term *purple-washing* to describe the tendency people have to gloss over, repress, or deny uncomfortable emotions, usually by "spiritualizing" the situation or by "being nice" about it. Purple-washers label certain emotions as "bad" and unacceptable and then fail to acknowledge them when they arise in the body. Purple-washers skip anger and go right to forgiveness; they push aside disappointment and say that "everything happens for a reason"; they skip jealousy and go right to feeling happy for people.

This glossing-over tendency is also referred to as *spiritual bypassing.* It's when we disconnect from emotions that we judge as bad or shameful, hop-stepping right over what's uncomfortable in our race to get to enlightenment and universal love. This tends to happen when we fixate our attention on the destination of our spiritual paths—pure compassion, love and light, bliss and oneness—rather than the real ups and downs of the path that's leading us there.

I have done my fair share of purple-washing in my lifetime. It took me until well into my twenties to even be able to recognize, let alone express, the emotion of anger in myself. I trace this back to my mother, who was a feisty Irish redhead. She was calm and loving most of the time, but when she got angry, she was *really* angry. My mother would do what I call a *stuff and blow:* She'd stuff her feelings away until she couldn't contain them anymore, at which point she would blow. When she got really angry, she would throw things. After my father had a massive stroke when I was ten, I never knew what was going to be flying around the house. Afterward, she'd act like nothing happened and she'd go right back to stuffing until she blew again. After witnessing many such episodes, I subconsciously decided that anger was bad and something I didn't want to feel.

I became very good at repressing not only anger but also fear. For the longest time, I could hardly recognize the emotion of fear in myself. In fact, fear was one of the last frequencies I learned to recognize in the field—which is rather strange, in hindsight, given that what I have found over the years of teaching is that fear is generally one of the easier emotions for students to detect, due to its pronounced and distinctive pulsing quality. A week or so after I heard it in a client, I was finally able to recognize the pulsing current of fear in myself. Circumstances of my childhood had apparently caused me to bury the experience of fear, and I had gone on to live, well, fearlessly. The first time I really recognized fear in myself was at a particular moment in my life when my husband and I were hanging by a thread financially, and the edge seemed awfully close. As I considered the ways things could play out, I suddenly became aware that the vibrational pattern traveling through my body was that pulsing feeling I had only recently identified in another person through the tuning forks. I was actually surprised and delighted to recognize it in myself, as strange as that sounds.

Then there's also *spiritual gaslighting:* the common tendency in conscious and wellness communities to blame oneself and others for not being able to maintain a "high vibration" state and consequently to manifest the life of one's dreams. If you're struggling with mental illness, having a crummy day, or stuck in a tough situation in your life—so the thinking goes—then your bad vibes and negative thinking must be the cause. This kind of thinking is yet another reason that I don't talk about "raising your vibration." While raising your vibration suggests overriding challenging emotions through forceful positive thinking, raising your voltage is about being fully embodied and present with whatever you are experiencing, and allowing all emotions to flow through without obstruction or suppression.

Many times, someone lying on my table has started to say, " I know I shouldn't feel this way, but . . ." Each time, I stop them right there. As human beings, we experience the full spectrum of emotions, whether we recognize them or not. Your emotions are important, all of them. There's nothing we "shouldn't" feel! And there is no such thing as a "negative" emotion. Every emotion is valid. Anger is not a negative emotion, it's a valid emotion. Rage is valid. Guilt is valid. We don't want to judge these emotions and tell them they're bad and have to go away. They're there for a reason. They're a part of the basic makeup of who we are, and they're a part of nature's perfect design.

I also love the way that the Human Design system describes emotions as a kind of navigation system designed to give us feedback about where we are on our path. This system nudges us along from that which is unhealthy and toward that which is healthy and appropriate for us. We lose this guidance system when our emotions are judged, avoided, and repressed. I like to think of them sort of like rumble strips on the side of the highway, letting us know when we've veered too far off course and are heading into the rough.

I invite you to ask yourself: Where do you draw the line within yourself between what's good and what's bad? How do you decide what's a positive emotion and what's a negative one? I love the saying "Life is like photography, we develop in the negative." It's cheesy, yes, but also very true. It is the difficulties and challenges in life that are our greatest catalysts for growth and expansion. Life has its ups and its downs, and sometimes the downs can feel *really* down. I find that the challenges tend to come in clusters, or what I call *shit storms*. When it rains, it storms! Whatever can go wrong seems to go wrong, and you end up with these really turbulent periods in your life. But when you come out the other side and you're able to reflect on it, what do you generally find? You've learned something. You've changed. You've grown. Once the dust settled, your life took a positive turn. Even when you've been handed some really difficult things, you rise to the occasion, you make it through, and you're a better person for it. Can you really say that an experience was "bad" if it changed your life in an ultimately positive way?

There's a visualization I use for helping people to really embrace the full range of human emotion. Just for a moment, close your eyes and contemplate all the waveforms in the universe. First, bring your awareness to the lowest imaginable waves that are thousands of light-years across from crest to trough. Contemplate the vastness of these low frequencies that travel in plasma through space. Then use your imagination to travel up the scale of frequency, allowing those waveforms to get a little bit shorter and closer together. Imagine them gradually becoming higher frequencies, but still vast and still below the audible range. Keep making them smaller and smaller, until they become the low tones of the audible range, and then move through the audible range up to the inaudible range. Then move up from there into the highest, finest frequencies that you can possibly imagine. Recognize that within your consciousness, you contain all of them: the infinite spectrum of sound, light, cosmic rays, gamma rays. You exist on every single one of those wavelengths. If you start getting too dialed in to any one particular waveform within yourself—whether it's anxiety or frustration or apathy or anything else—just acknowledge that. You don't have to deny it or push it away, but you can also open your mind and recognize that you're much more than that as well.

RIDING THE DRAGON

Once you're able to recognize and accept your emotions, then you need to figure out what you're going to do when the waves are breaking. How are you going to ride the wave? How are you going to use that energy?

Most people find that when they are finally able to release a backlog of emotion, they suddenly have reserves of energy to do things that they didn't have the energy to do before. The energy that was caught up in that stuck emotion suddenly becomes available for living and creating. We can channel that raw energy into something productive instead of letting it turn inward and become self-destructive. When you're angry, that's a powerful energy that you can use to get shit done! Anxiety, too, is an energy that wants to be expressed and channeled constructively. Clean your house, write in your journal, make a plan of action, get down and do some push-ups, take proactive steps toward changing what needs to be changed.

This process of harnessing our emotions into effective action is what

I call *riding the dragon*. I like to illustrate this process with the example of my then seventeen-year-old son, Cassidy. A while back, I went into Cassidy's bedroom to remind him that he had a dentist appointment that morning. Immediately, I felt the energy in the room start to churn with frustration and anxiety. It erupted from the bed and started swirling around his bedroom.

"Cassidy," I said, "you've gotta rein that shit in." I instructed him to get his clothes on and be ready to go in fifteen minutes.

"Mooooom!" he protested.

"Cassidy," I said flatly, "there's no room here for you to be an emotional wreck over going to the fucking dentist." I told him to harness those feelings and ride them out the door, because he needed to get his teeth cleaned. He admitted that I was right, got dressed, and got his butt over to the dentist on time.

If my teenage son can do it in these kinds of moments, anyone can. No matter how big or menacing the beasts of your emotions may feel in the moment, they are never bigger than you—unless you give them permission to be. You always have the choice to say, "I'm going to get it together and do what I need to do." There is a part of your mind that's alpha, and you have to decide to inhabit that part of yourself. When my students are working in someone else's field and start feeling overwhelmed when they encounter areas of intense turbulence, my response is always, "Breathe and ground like a boss!" Remember that you're in charge of your body, your mind, all your molecules and cells and electrical impulses. You are in control of yourself. Don't fall victim to your own stories of weakness telling you that you can't handle whatever's going on inside of you.

This is really about claiming our power and letting go of your stories of powerlessness. Ask yourself: What are the stories you're telling yourself about your emotions? Are you going to tell yourself a story of victimhood because that's your habit? Are you telling yourself that you're not in control, that there's nothing you can do? You can do that, but it's not necessary. Changing the narrative is as simple as changing your mind and deciding to adopt a new perspective. Our decisions carry great weight. Decide that you have the power and the ability to deal with whatever is arising in the moment.

That being said, there is a fine line between managing our emotions appropriately and moving through them, and purple-washing them. Where is that line? When do you give yourself space for something uncomfortable to surface, and when do you reel it in and get on top of it in an appropriate way? When are you yang, and when are you yin—and how do you know the difference between the two? Sometimes we need to just curl up and puddle in our emotions. Knowing when to puddle and when to ride the dragon out the door requires self-awareness. I've learned to tell the difference for myself by looking at my battery meter afterward—puddling at the right time can lead to a good bounce the next day, whereas forcing ourselves to power through may leave us even more exhausted and wrung out.

I don't want to be flippant when I talk about taking control of our emotions. There's some heavy stuff going on in the world and in many people's lives. I want to acknowledge those deeper wounds—experiences of unimaginable grief, of losing everything, being a victim of violence or hate crimes or institutionalized injustice. There are people who have gone through unspeakable pain and loss. If you lose a child or a spouse, that grief never goes away. Certain blows in life are more deeply imprinted than others. The wound of an abused or unmothered child is very deep. We have to acknowledge the reality of the pain body while at the same time seeking to get to a place beyond it. Certain things will never fully go away, but even then, we can still have moments when the soul feels free. We can still catch a glimpse of eternity in the eternal now. After many years of helping people heal, I believe that it is still possible to find a measure of joy and peace and gratitude even while the wounds still live inside of us.

CULTIVATING NEUTRALITY

Once the highs and lows of our emotions have passed, after the waves have risen and fallen, the mind returns to its neutral baseline. Neutrality is the place we return to once the highs and the lows have passed. It's a lovely place where there's no charge of happiness to maintain and no charge of sadness to wallow in or escape from. There is nothing to do, be, or accomplish here except simply to be present to our own experience of life. When we cultivate neutrality, we understand that life is full of ups and downs: good things and bad things happen because that is the nature of life. Life and emotions have their natural cycles and seasons. They rise and fall on their own in waves.

Cultivating neutrality is core to the work of managing our emotions. Neutrality isn't flatness or indifference. It's more like what Buddhists refer to as *equanimity*—the ability to experience life willingly and directly, without getting caught up in emotional reactions, and free from judgments of good and bad. Being at neutral means that you're not in a state of positive or negative charge. In fact, there's no emotional charge at all. You're neither happy nor sad, neither excited nor anxious, neither loving nor hating. You're not chasing after happiness or running away from pain and struggle. You simply *are*.

From a place of neutrality, we allow ourselves to feel our emotions as they arise, seeing that they are simply part of the universal human experience. We allow them to play out as they need to with a good laugh or a good cry or a brisk walk, or maybe some housecleaning or vigorous exercise if we're angry. We allow our emotions to run their course without judging or repressing them. Once the emotion has passed, we can simply allow ourselves to rest in that quiet, empty mental space and then be with whatever arises next. The more we are able to let our emotions flow, the more quickly we turn to the peace of neutrality.

Emotions—both the pleasant ones and the tough ones—ebb and flow. That is their nature. They're water element, not earth. What *can* be lasting is neutrality as a state of being that underlies those emotional waves. Learning how to bring yourself back to a neutral center over and over again is much more realistic than trying to be happy. Happiness is a spontaneous thing that arises when we experience a positive input. It generally goes away when the input is gone, or when a negative input takes its place, and that's perfectly okay! Life is not a lasting state of happiness or contentment or any other emotion. As the Buddhists have talked about ad nauseam, one of the greatest illusions of all is the illusion of permanence. This, too, shall pass.

A good trick for cultivating neutrality is to reframe the way you talk about your emotions. Have you ever noticed how people refer to their emotions differently in different cultures? In Germanic languages, like English and German, we refer to our emotions in terms of "being" them. *I am angry. I am sad. I am happy. I am ecstatic.* In Romance languages like French, Italian, and Spanish, people refer to their emotions in terms of "having" them: *I am having anger. I am having sadness. I am having happiness.* Now, if you compare Brits and Italians, who do you think is freer in their ability to express emotion? Take a page from the Italians' book and try shifting your language. Notice the difference in your inner experience when you *have* an emotion instead of *being* it. Is there a greater sense of detachment? Does the emotion pass through more quickly? Most people I've shared this with find the experience of *having* an emotion preferable to *being* it. It puts them back in that alpha part of their brain, and they can operate from a greater sense of control.

Now that we have a better understanding of our electromagnetic bodies and our emotions, we're going to take a journey into the biofield to look at how and where different emotions live in our fields and impact our bodies, and we'll explore what we can do to improve the way we interact with and manage them.

Part II

Your Biofield Anatomy

7

How to Work with Your Biofield

Emancipate yourself from mental slavery,
none but ourselves can free our minds

—Bob Marley

Your biofield is a map of your mind.

Whatever programs are running in your mind get mapped out in the electromagnetic field surrounding and interpenetrating your body. Over time, this creates energetic and physical patterns that our systems get stuck in, and as a result, we end up stuck in all these different areas of our lives: our physical health, our careers, and senses of purpose, relationships, finances, you name it. Any pattern in your life begins as a pattern in your energy field—in your mind.

We want to liberate ourselves from the patterns we've been stuck in so that we can find a greater sense of freedom and flow in our lives. Working on the level of the biofield gives us a direct way to access and to modulate those patterns, thereby redirecting the flow of energy in our systems.

Each chapter of Part II will focus on one of the main energy centers that we work with in Biofield Tuning: the feet, the knees, and the seven major chakras from the root to the crown. We will explore the particular set of emotions, mental patterns, and imbalances that I've identified in and around that particular energy center.

In addition to looking at the healthy, balanced expression of each energy center, we'll also explore the imbalances that occur when too much energy gets stuck out in the field on the left and right sides of that energy center. We're going to open up those right- and left-side file drawers to uncover the set of emotions, memories, and beliefs that have gotten frozen and sequestered in that particular part of the field. We'll be digging up the old files and deleting any programming that's not in service of our true potential, thereby liberating the data and battery power that were getting siphoned off into that faulty programming—and returning that energy to our neutral center and circulation, where it belongs. We'll also take a look at the back side expressions and what tends to occur when the backs of the chakras are closed off or weakened.

Some of this information will be familiar, and much of it will be new. The feedback I've received over the years is that the biofield anatomy offers a new perspective on the body and its underlying patterns, even for seasoned energy medicine practitioners. I encourage you to explore how my findings compare with, and complement, other systems of energy medicine. What I've discovered in mapping this relatively uncharted territory of the right, left, and back sides of the chakras is that there seems to be much more to learn about the chakras than what the ancient Vedic system—which remains the authority on the matter—originally documented.

I encourage you to meet everything you read here with a spirit of curiosity and skepticism. This is new terrain—for me, for you, and for our collective understanding of health and medicine. I am simply sharing my observations in the hopes that they will contribute to a greater understanding of our electromagnetic bodies that can help us to heal and thrive.

There's a universal challenge that those of us who work with Biofield Tuning face: The work is hard to explain, and often it's hard to believe. I spent years conducting sessions, wondering if what I was finding was real or if I was just making it up. It took me fifteen years before I really started to believe it—after I had logged over ten thousand hours of clinical research, written a master's thesis on the topic, and watched other people learn how to do it and find the same things I found—so if you're skeptical about all of this, that's quite okay! You should be. Nobody is more skeptical than I am. But after seeing this work benefit enough people, it's become clear to me that there is value in these discoveries. Truth is resonance. Take what resonates, and leave what doesn't. This is an evolving system that becomes stronger and more robust with every person who critically engages with it.

These patterns have proved, over the years, to be fairly universal. The same patterns have shown up in many thousands of Biofield Tuning sessions, conducted by me and the more than two thousand students who have been trained as of this writing. While I still find new and unexpected things in the field now and again, the core patterns haven't changed.

There are many more energy centers in the body than just the ones we'll be discussing. In addition to the seven major chakras, there are also minor energy centers throughout the body. I call these the *half steps,* and they include the high heart chakra, the diaphragm, the thighs, and the shins. Your major organs also contain their own minor energy centers. If you're interested in exploring the organs and half steps, I offer a range of recorded sessions on the Biofield Tuning website that target these areas.

WORKING WITH THE FIELD

I'm going to be teaching you how to use your own awareness like a tuning fork to detect and correct pockets of static, resistance, and stuck energy in your own biofield. While sound is a helpful tool, ultimately there is nothing more powerful than your mind. When it comes right down to it, you don't need anything beyond your awareness and intention to shift the flow of energy in your own system.

To work through any imbalances, stuck emotions, and faulty programming that you're encountering within your own field, I'll be offering coaching and tools that I've found to be helpful, including mantras and affirmations, visualizations, and suggestions for shifting your patterns of thought and behavior. These are tools that I use either during sessions to help move a client's energy or that I assign as "homework" to continue the work that a client has done in a session.

Whatever patterns you're working with, there are four key tools from the Biofield Tuning perspective that you can use to shift an unproductive pattern and get back to center: Activate your central channel; breathe, center, and ground; utilize the power of your mind; and utilize the power of sound.

ACTIVATE YOUR CENTRAL CHANNEL

A big key to electric health is having a strong current running through your central channel. This current of energy flow along your neutral midline also forms the outer boundary of your field. The energy of the central channel circulates out from the core, around the toroid, and back in again. This current flows bidirectionally, with the positive descending current and negative ascending current spiraling around each other. In addition to the centered presence that comes from a strong core, we also want that outer boundary to be really strong, because it helps protects us from the toxins and unbeneficial vibes in our environment.

I think of the central channel as our inner lightning rods. I start every Biofield Tuning session by activating the client's central channel. This is a way to strengthen their overall energy system and call their awareness back to the present moment. Start to think of yourself as an energetic torus and centralize your awareness in that neutral midline. Feel into the central channel that runs along your spine, from the center of your being all the way down into the center of the earth. By anchoring in our core, plumb and square in all our major energy centers, we come into electromagnetic alignment.

As we move through the field, we're collecting all the different pieces of ourselves from where they've been scattered and stuck and frozen, and we're bringing them back into that neutral midline, back into circulation, back to the present moment. The more of our energies that are tangled up out in the field, the more out of balance we become. When our central axis is tilting to the right or left sides of the field, we're not in the present moment. Our energies are tied up in the past, in our memories, our old stories, our "pain bodies." All our unprocessed and unintegrated experiences, everything we've ever experienced and even what our ancestors experienced, is encoded in the electromagnetic field surrounding our bodies. There's a lot of junk between us and the present moment. The doors of perception are pretty muddy!

Bringing your awareness back to the central channel is a key motion to be able to start to change your story and your stress response. Instead of getting triggered, you can come into electromagnetic alignment through the core of your being. When you're aligned in your central channel, you're doing what I call *surfing the now*. When we return to center, to the now, we're detaching from the old stories and the pain body. It's like stepping out of an old, heavy coat on a warm, sunny day. With that new sense of freedom and ease, we can start to let new stories and new possibilities come in.

As we explore the various right- and left-side imbalances, notice when your energy is getting off center and tilting to one side or the other. Much of what I do in Biofield Tuning is pulling people out of energetic ditches. I call the off-lying patterns on the right and left sides of the field the *left-hand ditch* and the *right-hand ditch*. While the central channel balances the masculine and feminine polarities (in Chinese medicine, the yin and yang), the right and left sides of the biofield hold the imbalanced, or excess, expression of masculine and feminine energy. The left-hand ditch holds the yin imbalances like sadness, disappointment, frustration, unmet needs and stifled expression, inertia and apathy, and powerlessness. The right-hand ditch holds the yang imbalances, which include anger, blame, aggression, overthinking and overdoing, and self-righteousness.

When our energies are stuck in a ditch, we become like a ship that's listing port or starboard. It always reminds me of when I was a coxswain on the crew team in prep school. The coxswain sits in back, steering the boat and coordinating the rhythm of the rowers. When we get stuck in frustration and disappointment, for example, it's like our energies start tilting left, to the port side of the boat. We're attaching into that old pattern of unmet needs, and the boat is starting to go off course. Whenever you become aware that you're drifting into the left-hand ditch, you can start to feel into the way that your energy is leaning to port. Notice what your inner alignment feels like. Or if you're stuck in anger and blame, imagine that you're listing to starboard, into the right-side ditch.

In these moments, you can choose to embody your inner coxswain and take control of where your ship is going. Coordinate your photons to shift that energy back to center. Recognize that you're attaching to an old pattern and you're getting all bunched up and off center in your sacral chakra, or wherever it might be. You can use your intention to detach your energy and awareness from wherever it's stuck in your field and bring that energy back into your neutral midline so you can use it to steer yourself where you want to go.

Over time, you'll start to develop the awareness to notice when your energy is getting all akimbo and zigzagged from old emotional patterns and stories. Whenever you become aware that you've drifted into a ditch, take a moment to reorient yourself. This is a basic mindfulness practice: Calling your energy back to center. Calling back, calling back, calling back your energy every time it drifts away and gets stuck somewhere it's not supposed to be. Feel into your core, and feel your connection to ground. Rest in electromagnetic equilibrium between heaven and earth. Reel yourself back in. This energy shift only takes a minute, and you can repeat it as many times as you need.

Fundamentally, we are not looking to be "happy" per se, but rather resting in the contentment that naturally arises from successfully settling into the neutral now. This state of ease allows the body to function optimally.

BREATHE, CENTER, AND GROUND

Learning how to breathe is a critical part of this work. Breath *is* energy, plain and simple. It's pure life force. Without the breath, you are not alive. Without breath, your battery will die within minutes. And remember, you're not just breathing in oxygen, you're also breathing in electricity. At every moment, you breathe in plasma, charged particles, light, and movement. We can go for weeks without food, days without water, but only minutes without breath. Not only does the breath provide us with energy, we can also use the breath to *move* and *discharge* energy.

But we've lost this basic knowledge of how to breathe freely. Most people breathe up in their chests rather than all the way down into their bellies, and as a result, they don't fully occupy their own bodies. When we have emotions that we don't want to feel and we don't want to deal with, we don't allow the breath to flow there, because *we* don't want to go there. This happens more than anything else with the really uncomfortable emotions like anger, powerlessness, guilt, and shame that lurk in our bellies and lower digestive tracts. When you start breathing again, the emotions start to come up and release. That might not feel great, because the emotions are uncomfortable, but the release is what liberates the energy back into flow.

In my group sessions, I act as a channel for the energies of the group. As I encounter places of dissonance and stuckness, it causes me to tighten up and not breathe. Whenever that happens, I know that other people aren't breathing, because my body is resonating with the energy of the group. If you ever listen to one of my recorded sessions, you'll hear me audibly exhale at many points throughout the sessions, because that's how I'm discharging the group's energy.

We want to locate those places of tension that cause us to hold our breath subconsciously. This work is going to help you to relax these places and all these subconscious inputs or difficult life stories that have caused us to tense up and to tighten and to not breathe and that block life force. As you're reading and you encounter trigger points of tension in your field that cause you to restrict your breath, you can release that tension through a deep exhale. In fact, take a nice deep breath right now! Whenever you feel your breath tightening, notice any places that feel locked, stuck, or dark in your body. See if you can breathe into those places. If you're having trouble getting into your body and you feel stuck in your thoughts, ask yourself:

- What is it in my body that I'm avoiding?
- Why am I dissociating from my feeling sense?
- What's uncomfortable in my system right now? Can I breathe into that?

With your breath, bring awareness to the tension, and use your intention to consciously let it go. Visualize your electric circuitry and imagine liquid golden light going into that place instead.

A practice we use in Biofield Tuning is the centering and grounding breath. You simply breathe into your belly, deep into the area behind and below your navel. On the exhale, use your intention to direct the breath down and out your tailbone, or down your legs and out through your feet. We're centering by bringing the breath deep into the belly, and we ground by consciously sending that energy down. This is a grounding breath that discharges the energy through the tailbone or feet. It takes the tension and sends it into the ground. This breath helps discharge your vagus nerve—the long nerve that connects your brain to your heart and all your other organs. When you get tense, it bunches up. To release it, we use our breaths to take that tension and send it down into the ground. (We'll also talk about other ways to ground your energy in the next chapter on the feet centers.)

USE YOUR MIND: AWARENESS AND INTENTION

You can be the tuning fork and learn to use your mind to move your inner photonic arrangement through awareness.

Energy follows thought. What we put our focus on, grows. What we neglect, declines. We can use our knowledge of this principle to shift and redirect the flow of energy in our system. The mind is a powerful thing! Power, I think, is really just understanding that you are a magnetic being and that you have the ability to impact the magnetic field—both your individual electromagnetic field and the collective field—through the use of your mind.

There are a few key ways to use your mind to shift patterns of energy flow. The first is to increase your awareness by simply identifying what's present. As things are coming up to be processed, name what you're finding in clear, neutral terms. This is something I do in every Biofield Tuning session, especially in groups. I'll hit a patch of distortion in the field and share the vibrational information that I'm reading, whether it's a lack of nurturing in early childhood, a story of unworthiness, a fear of being seen, or a buildup of unexpressed creative energy.

So much of what we're doing is simply bringing these emotions and energetic structures to light. When I name something—especially something that doesn't seem to be budging even after repeated forays into it—that thing gets brought to light. Sometimes just shining a light on the pattern is sufficient to get it to clear. We're able to take that emotion or experience out of the basement of the subconscious mind where it's been hiding and examine how it's been affecting us. Then, once we're conscious of the pattern, we can choose whether or not to continue it. That's not a "one and you're done" choice. Those subconscious currents can still continue to derail us despite our best intentions, especially the strong ones. It takes a continual discipline to override strongly ingrained patterns.

When something needs a bit more cajoling, I turn to affirmations and visualizations to use the power of intention to help shift the energy. An affirmation ("I am open to the possibility of seeing things differently") is simply a declaration of an intention. An affirmation like "I am in control of my finances," spoken with conviction and positive feeling, can quickly shift a fear pattern around money. It's incredible how a fork stuck in a pocket of energy that's thick as molasses will start to move effortlessly when the individual repeats an affirmation with real force of intention behind the words. I offer many affirmations throughout the text, and you can also come up with your own based on your particular intention.

Other times, I use visualizations to shift the flow of energy. I will guide people through a process of visualizing and removing a block, wall, or other constraining object, like a ball and chain, from some part of their fields. What we can imagine has a certain reality—not only in mind but in matter. Studies have shown that mental practices like imagining oneself lifting weights results in actual increases in muscle mass and in some cases can be almost as effective as physical exercise. If you can shift patterns in your physiology using your imagination, don't you think you should be able to shift your energy and emotions in the same way?

Try the affirmations and visualizations I've provided, notice any shifts in your energy that occur, and get creative in making up your own. I have done my best to make all my exercises and suggestions simple and easy to do, as I am one of those people who tends to gloss over the exercise parts of books, especially if they are complicated! The most important thing is to fully engage with these ideas and apply whatever new awareness you gain in the context of your everyday life.

UTILIZE THE POWER OF SOUND

I am going to talk a lot about Biofield Tuning because it's been the pathway and the process that led me to the information about how to improve your electric health, that provided me with the insight to better understand and make use of our amazing human minds and bodies. But there are a ton of other great modalities out there that utilize sound if you're interested in working with sound healing.

And there are a million different ways to tap into the power of sound on your own! You can use your voice and create harmonious resonance in your body through humming, toning, singing, whistling, or chanting. The biggest thing that got me through the grief of losing my mother when I was twenty-five was listening to music and singing at the top of my lungs.

Music is powerful medicine. It is arguably the most effective healing tool that you can access at pretty much any time, often free of cost. Start listening to different types of music consciously with the intention of shifting your energy and your emotional state. Put on music while you work or clean. Learn an instrument. I am learning to play the electric guitar at the moment (at fifty-one!), and it is a great meditation because you can't be thinking while you are playing. Singing in groups has been scientifically documented to boost immunity and spirits. The longest-living occupation is musical conductor, who are bathed in coherent sound all the time!

If you have a tuning fork, you can use it to feel into and harmonize with your emotions. If you're feeling angry, try putting a tuning fork on your liver. If you're feeling scared, try resting the handle of the fork on your kidneys. You can purchase a 128 Hz weighted tuning fork for under ten dollars online and start playing around. While that kind of fork isn't the quality of what we use in sound therapy work, it will allow you to start exploring. If you're interested in investing in higher-quality forks, I recommend starting with the Sonic Slider, my most popular fork. It's available online at the Biofield Tuning store.

The vibrational power of words is also a part of the story of sound. When you repeat mantras or affirmations, you're tapping into the power of intention and the power of sound at the same. In each chapter, I've included the Vedic seed syllable mantras (also known as *bija mantras*) that are connected with each chakra. In Sanskrit, *mantra* means an "instrument of mind" or "instrument of thought." The seed syllables are said to activate the energy of the chakras, and when used as a mantra, they become an instrument for attuning your mind to the vibration of a particular chakra. Listen to these mantras, repeat them aloud, or even better, make a meditation out of chanting the mantra for ten to fifteen minutes while centering your awareness in that particular energy center and "tuning" yourself to its frequency.

Our chakras are transponders of sound and light waves, and as such, each chakra has a particular range of the electromagnetic spectrum that it is correlated with—represented by a color and a vowel sound. (Some people also correlate the chakras with the notes of the Western musical scale, something I did with tuning forks at the beginning of my practice but no longer do.) Each chapter will mention the color and vowel sound associated with that particular chakra. Get creative with using the power of color and sound to connect with the unique frequencies of your various energy centers. I recommend humming or toning the vowel sound while sending the vibration to that part of your body.

If you're not familiar with vocal toning, it is the practice of producing a steady tone (like "ahh" or "eeee") with your voice while exhaling, and it is believed to harmonize and balance the body's energetic channels. I have certainly found it to be effective for getting stuck energy flowing again, and I have asked clients to tone many times during Biofield Tuning sessions. Especially when working on the throat chakra, toning is an excellent tool for opening up the vocal pathways and creating greater resonance in the body.

HEALING, FAST AND SLOW

Discovering and digesting the unresolved emotions in your biofield is going to take some time and care and curiosity. A lot of people come to Biofield Tuning (or any other kind of healing work) looking for the big breakthrough, but it's not a "flip the switch and you're done" kind of thing. One or two sessions can create dramatic changes in some people, but the real work of continuing the journey needs to come from the individual themselves. It is the way they integrate the work in their lives that matters most. When we're looking for the quantum leap, we often refrain from putting one foot in front of the other and taking it one step at a time.

Certain aspects of the healing journey require us to settle in for the long haul. Real self-mastery takes time. It takes trying and failing, falling off, and getting back on again and again. It's like becoming a better sailor. You just have to get out there and put your sails up and learn. Achieving mastery with anything is a long-term commitment, and mastery with mind and emotions is no different. I don't think it should take you the thirty years it took me to figure all this out, so I'm giving you tools that I've found to be effective in speeding the process. But it's not an "I'll start on Monday" thing. We deal with every pattern, every problem, in the proper time.

It's a commitment to your own well-being and a consistent discipline over your own mind that creates change over time. But it doesn't have to be a drag! It can be fun. I highly recommend gamifying even the most challenging aspects of your life. Thinking of it all as a video game can help us to stay in a place of neutrality and presence. You're just moving through all these different levels of the game, and meanwhile, you have to keep your health meter and your wealth meter up so that you can overcome obstacles and keep advancing through the levels.

Keep coming back to center. Be a creative problem-solver. Adapt and overcome. Enjoy the game. Celebrate the moments when you level up.

8

FEET: The Ground You're Standing On

One of my personal problem areas has been my feet. I've suffered with pain, plantar warts, athlete's foot, fallen arches, and a strange sense of general disconnection with my feet. My left foot has been particularly challenging. When I trained my first group of students in 2010 and I started to get worked on for the first time, my students and I were both aghast at the atonality around my left foot. Truly, it sounded worse than anything I had ever heard on anyone.

"How can you seem so 'together' but sound so awful?" one of my students asked me.

"Compartmentalization," I replied. "I am very good at it!"

It was true. I had learned to seal off all the broken, wounded, sad, hurting, angry bits of myself and construct a highly functional part of me that was able to soldier through despite being disconnected from a large portion of my body and my mind.

At the time, I had seven plantar warts on my left foot that no attempts to remove had been successful. Clearly, my immune system had abandoned that zone of my body, just as my own mind had. There was too much pain, discomfort, suffering, and unhappiness present there—a familiar feeling set during childhood that continued throughout my life as I seemed to be continually immersed in challenging situations that I could not extract myself from. Somewhat miraculously, the plantar warts disappeared after just a few tunings (other clients have also reported this, so it is not out of the norm), and my life slowly began to change direction as it dawned on me that constant struggle didn't have to be inevitable.

In the biofield anatomy, the feet have to do with our ability to take our next steps in life. When we're struggling, for whatever reason, to move away from that which isn't serving us and toward that which does, it shows up as distortion and blockage in the energy centers around our feet. Each foot contains distinct energy and information. While the left foot represents where we're coming from (and what we might be stuck in), the right foot speaks to me of where we're headed next. The answers to questions like *Where are you going? How are you getting there? What is the ground that you're standing on? What is your path in life? How do you feel about your life right now?* can all be found in the record of information stored in the magnetic field surrounding and interpenetrating the feet.

It's no coincidence that I ended up with a colony of warts on my left foot. When we withdraw our awareness from a part of our body-mind, we also withdraw life-giving energy and the intelligence of the immune system. It just doesn't go there, because there is a wall in the mind that says, "We don't go here." But the body will find a way to let us know that there is a problem somewhere that needs to be addressed, even if our conscious mind has cleverly tucked it away. The body starts jumping up and down, saying, "Excuse me! There's a problem here. Please take a look." It will create symptoms to draw our attention to the energetic imbalance—from mild discomfort all the way to disease and injury—so that we can do what needs to be done to fix it. Often, our awareness is enough to kick-start the healing process.

THE FEET IN THE BIOFIELD ANATOMY

In addition to the seven major chakras, or energy centers, I discovered early on that there were also minor energy centers in our feet and knees. We don't have a very good understanding of these energy centers, and as a result, they don't tend to get a whole lot of attention. But what I've found is that they play a crucial role in our overall health and well-being. If we want to have a healthy energy system with optimum voltage running through our wires, it's critical to address the energetic health of the feet and knees.

I'll admit that I was perplexed by the feet for a long time. It took many years of work to even begin to figure them out. The problem is that I was getting so much data that I couldn't quite narrow it down. The feet contain a great deal of complex information. In a certain way, everything is contained in the feet, and that's what I was feeling. You can do a tuning session on someone's entire body just by working on their feet.

Many ancient medicinal traditions (including in India, Egypt, and China) viewed the feet as a reflection of one's general state of being, so it makes sense that we would encounter so many different kinds of experiences, emotions, thought structures, and memories here. In Chinese medicine, the feet (like the hands and ears) are seen as a microcosm of the system as a whole, containing a map of the body in its entirety.

Over time, the picture that emerged from all the data I was taking in revealed that the feet were strongly related to the metaphorical "ground beneath our feet." The vibrations present in the feet began to speak to me of the path that someone had walked for decades (and perhaps even lifetimes), as well as the direction they were heading in. They also spoke of the emotions, beliefs, and thought patterns that person carried around their ability to move forward on their life path.

In their healthy and balanced expression, each foot supports us in walking in the direction of our dreams, desires, and highest growth. A healthy right foot allows us to boldly move forward in the direction of our dreams, to take action and risks, to have clarity around decisions, and to get out of our comfort zones and step into the unknown. With a healthy left foot, we are able to leave behind situations and environments (which could be either internal or external) that we've felt stuck or trapped in. When the left foot is on line and coherent, we recognize our biological impetus to walk away from something that's not good for our health, our energies, our relationships, or our happiness and toward something that will better serve us.

What we call *life* is nothing more than our journeys through this earth plane and the steps we take along the way. And to move confidently in the right direction, we need the support of healthy and strong foot energy. Think about the ground you're standing on right now and how your feet are supporting and uplifting you along the path of your life. *Where are your feet? Where are you stepping? Are you walking or running or dancing? Are you trudging along? Are you fighting an uphill battle?* In so many people's feet, I find the programming of "uphill battle, uphill battle, uphill battle." That energy creates a very distinct tone in the forks. It's a vibration of struggle and difficult characters and rocky roads.

It takes a tremendous amount of bravery to be free in the feet. What we're really talking about here is the freedom to follow the call of your soul, wherever that might lead. To do that, you have to trust in yourself, in the universe, and in God or spirit or the unified field or whatever else you want to call it. We have to trust enough to be willing to step out of our "known zones" and into the "great unknown" of our own unique paths, which is never linear or predictable. That takes big courage—both to step away from that which is not serving us and also to step into that which we truly desire.

GROUNDING AND DISCHARGING

Healthy feet also support our basic grounding and embodiment in physical reality, our ability to stand tall and strong with our "feet on the ground," so to speak. When the energy of the feet is blocked or distorted, we find ourselves drifting around with our heads in the clouds, disassociated from our bodies and environment.

One key function of a healthy foot chakra is allowing energy that's passed through the system and is no longer needed to be released from the body and recycled back into the earth. If the foot chakras are open, energy passes through freely and consistently. This allows us to be in energetic equilibrium with the environment. It's a whole lot easier to feel grounded when our energies are circulating properly and discharging through the feet.

Think back to your toroidal biofield: the ascending and descending streams of energy, what the yogic tradition calls the *Ida* and *Pingala,* are continuously flowing up and down the central channel. The role of grounding is to keep that flow of energy moving in both directions. Through the feet, we release the descending (positively charged) energy that's made its way through the system down into the earth and simultaneously soak up fresh new life force (negatively charged) from the ground beneath us.

If your foot chakras are weakened or congested, that process of release is thwarted. Instead of passing through and out the feet, the energy just recirculates back up into the higher energy centers, creating a backlog of excess electrostatic energy in the body, which builds up over time and creates inflammation.

There are so many things in our inner and outer environments that load us up with excess electromagnetic charge, from incoherent thoughts and emotions to Wi-Fi signals to chemical exposure. Taking care of our electrical health means learning to discharge this excess energy, and the process of releasing energy through the feet and into the earth is the most important way we naturally do that.

A good way to ground your energy is to stimulate the Kidney 1 (K1) point on the bottom of each foot. In Biofield Tuning, we begin every session by activating the K1 point using the weighted tuning forks. As the lowermost energy point on the body in Chinese medicine, it's often used in acupuncture and acupressure to ground a patient's energy and drain excess energy from the head, neck, and shoulders. The Chinese name for this point translates to "Gushing Spring," which gives you a sense of how powerfully it can release energy. I've found K1 to be an excellent grounding point. Simply rub the K1 point on each foot with a strong hand for thirty to sixty seconds in the morning or at night to ground and clear your energy body. Eden Energy Medicine uses the technique of rubbing a spoon on that spot to accomplish the same thing, so that is also an option. Bonus points if you want to add a visualization: I like to imagine activating the winged feet of the messenger god Mercury. Having those wings on our feet can help us to be fleet-footed and to change direction with ease.

My personal approach to grounding is being barefoot or wearing leather-soled shoes and earthing, or grounding (being in direct contact with the earth's surface), whenever I can. Rubber-soled shoes prevent electric energy from moving in and out of the feet, so we end up with that excess of energy that creates inflammation. Whatever the body is trying to release is bouncing off the soles of our shoes and back up into our bodies. Rubber is an insulator, so not only does it block the flow of electrons coming up from the earth, it also halts the flow of protons, the positive flow that descends through the body from above the crown. When we connect to ground (either barefoot, ideally, or in leather-soled shoes), we're sending that ascending energy into the earth and then pulling up the negative energy through K1 so that our feet have a balanced positive and negative charge.

When I first started the practice of grounding by walking barefoot in a grassy park for about thirty minutes each day, I was astonished at how much better it made me feel. All these years, I had been trying this diet and that gadget and this program, and nothing had been as simple, easy, or effective as just taking off my shoes! I slept better, my gums stopped bleeding, and my energy levels went way up.

I'm telling you right now: Getting rubber-soled shoes out of your life can do wonders for reducing anxiety and inflammation. I preach the virtues of leather-soled shoes at every chance I get! But the important thing is just to get your feet on the ground somehow, and to do it as much as you can. Stand on the grass in your local park, go barefoot in your backyard, or let your feet out for a walk in the countryside. If it is too cold, you can hug trees (really) or just use your imagination very clearly, expanding your field out and into the ground. Get connected to the ground in whatever way is easiest for you.

RIGHT FOOT: LEAVING THE "KNOWN ZONE"

I call the right foot the "leap of faith" foot. Becoming free in the right foot (and also the right knee) is about allowing ourselves to recognize and follow the soul's true path, wherever it might lead. What is it that prevents you from running in the direction of your dreams and doing all the beautiful things that your soul is calling you to do? Fear is almost always the answer. That is the number-one programming that gets stuck in the right foot and prevents us from taking our next steps in life.

Fear is a very strong signal jammer. It has a pulsating frequency that tends to block out other signals—meaning, it overrides other thoughts and emotions. You can find the frequency of fear pretty much anywhere in the biofield, depending on what kind of experience is giving rise to it, but the area around the right foot is one of the main places where fear builds up and creates a signal jam. It is also a frequency that is very easy to recognize, if you know what you're looking for, and it's usually one of the first emotions that my students are able to correctly identify.

In the right foot in particular, we're typically dealing with the fear of the unknown. The fear of leaving one's "known zone" is a programming encoded deep in our nervous systems that can often be traced all the way back to birth. Being born is itself a transition. If that transition was painful and traumatic—as it is for many people—then on a deep level, we will hold the belief that transitions are painful. That belief creates a deep fear of taking our next steps and moving boldly into new territories.

When we experience painful transitions, whether it's birth, a sudden or jarring change in family life during childhood, a big move, or an unwelcome change of job or relationship, it creates a tremendous fear of the consequences of taking our next steps. Your nervous system goes into hypervigilance and will tell you that any movement into the unknown is going to bring hurt. *It's not safe.* And what makes us feel safe or unsafe plays a *huge* role in what we choose to do. If your parents passed away when you were a child and you had to leave your home and move in with your grandparents, later in life, leaving the "home" of your known zone is going to trigger a huge amount of fear and trepidation. Even if the known sucks, the voice of fear tells us that the unknown might suck even more. We decide to stay with the *familiar* fear instead of confronting the *unfamiliar* fear that might lead to our growth or liberation or expansion.

Fear is not bad. We're not trying to get rid of it. Fear about taking a leap is normal and appropriate. And contrary to what some people might think, that fear never really goes away. If you're waiting for the fear to go away before you take whatever step the universe is nudging you toward, you're never going to go anywhere. You'll never grow or expand in the ways your soul is calling you to. All that unexpressed energy and life force that wants to leap into the unknown will get frozen and tucked away in a little pocket in the lower right-foot corner of your field.

Fear is the body's way of saying, "This is new, and I don't know what's coming. I need to pay attention." You need that vigilance! But you don't need paralyzing fear. There's fear in motion, and then there's frozen fear. Rather than getting rid of the fear, we want to put it in motion. When we move into action, that fear begins to shift into excitement. The awareness alone that we can live with fear and accept it without having it paralyze us already creates a shift.

Those of us who are risk takers constantly take steps that are scary, but we've concluded that the discomfort of the known is more uncomfortable than the discomfort of the risk and expansion. I have found that people who experience a lot of fear around taking risks often had parents who frequently yelled or snapped at them for "doing something wrong." When that happens, you can become traumatized around taking action. You begin to associate taking risks with being punished, so you go into inertia mode. But it's deeply subconscious. We want to flex the "taking action" muscle and align our consciousness with it. If that muscle is flabby and underutilized, you can make it strong through regular, small repetitions. You don't make a muscle strong by going from zero to bench-pressing hundreds of pounds. You start with just a few minutes a day of biceps curls with a two-pound weight and you work your way up. With very little pain or discomfort, the muscle gets stronger.

The trick is to feel the fear, acknowledge it, recognize it, and muster the courage to leap anyway. And if you're not even sure where you're being called to take a leap, your friend fear will tell you exactly where. You can actually use the frequency of fear as a sonar pointing you in the direction of where your soul is calling you to stretch and expand. When you feel disconnected from your magnetic sense, or you've gotten so used to ignoring your internal nudges that you can't even hear them anymore, the louder voice of fear will tell you exactly where you're being called to step into the unknown.

I have been repeatedly terrified by the things the universe has nudged me to do, but I've learned to trust these nudges and do it anyway. When the universe says, "Jump," I jump, no matter how scared I am in that moment. To me, that is the secret of living the life of your dreams.

Fear can also show up as indecision. We are afraid to make the wrong choice, so we waffle back and forth, but fail to jump. One thing to keep in mind around indecision is this: Very often if you can't decide, you either don't have enough information or the answer is neither of your options (or maybe both!). When we know, we know, and it is something we determine with our guts, not our hearts or brains.

I recently twisted my right ankle while walking across ice, something that I am usually very good at avoiding, because my system is generally resilient and responsive. However, I had spent the previous few months uncharacteristically wavering on two big decisions with my business: Do I do this or that? Which direction do I move forward in? That energetic dithering created a weakness in the field around my foot, making it less responsive and able to stop the twist, and the resulting injury really flared and forced me to look at how painful that process, and one decision in particular, had been. Once I acknowledged what was going on in my mind and my emotions (as well as used the Sonic Slider on it), the pain and swelling somewhat miraculously disappeared in just a few hours.

LEFT FOOT: STUCK OR MIRED IN TOXIC SITUATIONS

As much as we need courage to step boldly into the unknown, we also need it to step away from the situations in our lives that *aren't* working for us.

The left foot speaks to our ability to walk away from toxic or unproductive people, places, or circumstances. When I'm working in the field around someone's left foot, I often feel a sense of being stuck in a unbeneficial situation that's been familiar to the person for years, decades, or longer. I call this being *mired*. The field off the left foot gets very charged up when we are stuck in these kinds of situations. That could be all sorts of things, from living in a big city when we yearn to be closer to nature, to staying with an abusive partner. When we want to pull away from something that's toxic or stressful, but we feel that we can't, the energy that the body wants to mobilize to walk away instead gets frozen and sequestered around the left foot.

The horrific tone of my own left foot had to do with a lifetime history of being a people pleaser and getting stuck in situations that worked for those around me but didn't work for me. I didn't have good boundaries, I absorbed other people's pain, my self-care was abysmal, and I was under perpetual emotional stress because of it. Once I started getting tunings and becoming more aware of the patterns, I saw that the warts on my left foot spoke of the denial I was in regarding my continual discomfort, to the point of my immune system not being able to even recognize or address these viruses that had taken up residence here. Especially as women, we often allow ourselves to stay in uncomfortable situations that are familiar for the sake of others. We end up compromising, accommodating, and selling ourselves short because we've been programmed and conditioned to take care of everyone else before ourselves, and I was no exception.

An image that often comes to mind in sessions is a shackle around the left ankle. Think about when a baby elephant is being trained: they put chains and shackles on their back leg and stake them into the ground so that they can't go anywhere. That's how the elephant is trained to act a certain way and to override its own free will. Then when the elephant is an adult, and the chain gets replaced by a flimsy rope, it won't run away, because it's been conditioned to believe that it can't go anywhere. That's a pretty good metaphor for what's going on in the left foot for many of us. There's a feeling of being imprisoned in an uncomfortable or unhealthy situation, along with an inability to recognize that now, as adults, we can engage our free will to move away from these stressors.

This programming is deeply rooted when we're born into a vibration of toxicity in our environment. As babies and children, we don't have the option to leave, and we are forced to adapt to the toxicity. Our consciousness disconnects from the situation because it's too painful or uncomfortable, but the emotions stick around, ultimately freezing up in the field around the left foot. Instead of recognizing the toxic influence and trying to step out of it and toward something healthier, we simply go numb because that is the established pattern.

A big part of what keeps people mired in toxic situations is a fear of the consequences if they try to escape. But what I observe more often is that it's the person's stories of helplessness that are keeping them stuck. If you were stuck in a toxic home environment as a child and had no ability to walk away, you start telling yourself stories that reinforce a sense of powerlessness and victimhood. It's a very deep programming that tells us that we're doomed, we'll never get out, we'll never fix it, things will never change. When we're adults, those stories might show up as the voice of: "It's hard," "I can't," "I don't have the money/time/energy," "I guess it will always be this way." This often creates a low, buzzy tonal quality indicating a sense of sadness, apathy, and inertia.

I once had a woman in one of my classes who had what felt like an energetic moon boot around her left foot. Her life was an ongoing story of being mired in bad situations. She was the product of an accidental pregnancy, and she was born to parents who didn't love each other and didn't want her. As an adult, she found herself in a loveless marriage and had strained relations with her children. She never walked away from any of the toxic situations in her life because she felt stuck there, just as she'd been stuck as a child in a loveless home. The lifelong belief that she had no power over situations that didn't work for her and were hurting her created a pocket of massive resistance that sucked in all the energy around it.

During her session, we were able to clear up and shift that pattern, and that evening after class, she went back to the Airbnb where she had been staying. But as soon as she got in, she said to herself, *You know what? I really don't like this place. I don't feel comfortable here.* Although she'd felt uncomfortable from the get-go, it was the first moment she recognized that she actually had a choice to leave, whereas the day before, she felt obligated to stay because she'd already paid for it, she didn't want to be rude, and so on. But without that moon boot around her foot, she felt the *freedom* she needed to make a different choice and act on it. She packed up her things, checked into a nice hotel where she felt more comfortable, and was able to get the most out of the training.

Her situation is not unusual. So many of us subconsciously endure bullshit for the simple reason that *we believe we have to*! It doesn't even dawn on us that we might have another option. We've completely blinded ourselves to the potential solutions. But once the energy of the left foot comes back on line, the aperture of possibility and potential opens up. Suddenly, we start to see other choices. This is growth! This is healing. It's when new choices and alternatives appear in our awareness, and we're able to freely act on them.

Our stories of victimhood aren't nearly as powerful as we make them out to be. When I encounter the tone of a victim story in the field, I'll tell the person what I'm experiencing in as much detail as I can. Just in hearing someone else speak it and identify it, their energy already starts to shift. There's often a "Hell no!" response when the person realizes that they've been telling themselves that they're powerless to help themselves and change their lives. The alpha part of ourselves takes over and says, "I'm not going to continue to make myself a victim. I'm taking control."

There's a powerful visualization I often use to help people remove an energetic ball and chain from their feet. Sit in silence for a moment, breathing deeply and drawing your attention inward. Call to mind an area of your life where you've felt stuck in old patterns and afraid to move forward. Imagine this fear of the unknown as a ball and chain attached to your left foot that you're breaking out of so that you can walk forward without that weight holding you back. Then, allow yourself to feel what it feels like to be unbound from all the things that bind you, all the things that keep you from moving confidently toward that which you desire— the debt, the excess weight, the self-doubt, the business failure. What would it *feel like* if those things just suddenly fell away? Imagine the lock of the chain unlocking, and see yourself walking forward, free from that weight pulling you down. Stay with this feeling of freedom and confidence for a few minutes and call upon it freely in your day whenever you start to feel bogged down.

You are the only one who can free yourself from these stories of victimhood and powerlessness. Healing is detaching from your old stories, from the things you keep telling yourself over and over again, and opening to a new story. Ask yourself: What is the chapter you want to close? What is the old story of stuckness and powerlessness? Nature doesn't tolerate a vacuum; to get rid of the old story, you need to replace it with a new one. What does chapter 2 look like? Who are you in your new story?

9

KNEES: Getting Unstuck

The knees were the last part of the biofield I ever started working on. When I got my first set of tuning forks back in 1996, there were seven forks with the tones C, D, E, F, G, A, and B, accompanied by a little instruction booklet that told you which fork to use on which chakra. With the booklet as my guide, that's exactly what I did: I went up through the chakras with the different forks, starting at the tailbone with the root chakra and ending at the top of the head with the crown chakra.

This simple process worked well, but I kept finding that after I finished a session, my clients were leaving feeling somewhat light-headed and dazed. I started using the forks on the feet to ground the person's energy at the end of a session. That did the trick. Then one day, years later, as I was tuning a woman's feet at the end of her session, it occurred to me for the first time that perhaps I should try working on the field of her knees. This was something that had never even occurred to me before. So I gave it a try, and my immediate reaction was . . . "Oh, dear!" I couldn't believe how much "stuff" I found there. And it wasn't just her. As I began experimenting on the knees, I found that almost every single person who was showing up on my table had a significant amount of dissonance and blockage in their knees. This was a serious omission on my part! I'd been skipping over an entire energy center—and one, I would learn, that plays a highly overlooked role in our overall health and well-being.

What I discovered over time was that the information in the knees seemed to reveal the degree of inner and outer freedom a person was experiencing in their lives. With strong and healthy knees, we are free to follow our natural inclinations. We move and act spontaneously. The healthy tone of the knees is so relaxed and confident. It's an easygoing, fluid power with an almost serpentine and sensual feel to it. Think about the graceful movements of a downhill skier or snowboarder—that's the power and agility of the knees. In traditional yogic practices, there's a huge emphasis on knee mobility (think: lotus pose). To free their minds, ancient yogic masters engaged in vigorous training to open up and extend the range of motion of their knees.

When our knees are free, we can use them to direct ourselves this, that, and the other way. We move our bodies and lives in the direction that our spirit is pointing us, at the appropriate speed for ourselves and our present needs. We are able to engage in what I call *spontaneous appropriate action*. What that looks like is allowing yourself to be moved in the moment. The universe moves through us. It's almost like dancing. You're moving through life responding to the music and movements of other dancers, rather than repeating the same old stories and knee-jerk emotional reactions rooted in past experiences and traumas. You're able to progress in your life with trust, without needing to control or overplan the future. You flow freely with the current of life. Spontaneous appropriate action is about *improvising* rather than needing to follow a script. That spontaneity often moves us toward play, lightness, and creative expression.

The blocked or imbalanced expression of the knees is stuckness—the opposite of freedom and spontaneity. When the energy of the knees isn't flowing, we can't seem to do what we need to do to get where we're trying to go in our lives. In the right knee, I find obstacles or challenges moving forward, while the left knee contains information related to trust around letting go of the devil you know versus staying in habits and situations that we would be better off growing out of.

The backs of the knees hold issues relating to clarity and certainty. When people swell up in the backs of their knees, it's usually an indication that they are stuck in uncertainty about something, not knowing if they should go this way or that way. The knee chakras, and our energy systems as a whole, end up suffering greatly from that energy of not knowing what to do.

The knees, like the feet, are holographic in nature. They contain information related to the whole body. Each knee is an entry point for information contained throughout the system related to obstacles moving forward. An issue that I find in the knees might have a correlation in the throat, for instance, if the obstacle is a suppression of creativity or self-expression, or perhaps in the third eye if there's a lack of clarity around our deeper purpose that is preventing us from taking our next steps.

When there's a lot of static and interference around the knees, any attempt to move forward into our own flow and to get out of the places where we've been stuck is also blocked. Imagine if you put someone in cement up to their knees—that's pretty much what it feels like to have an energetic backlog in the knees. If your knees are locked up, you're not going anywhere! Instead of flowing, we stagnate. We stop being able to move in new ways.

If you think of your electrical circuitry, energy moves along established pathways. Instead of moving creatively, we default to these grooves that are already well worn. The neural circuitry of old thought patterns is already established, and that's where the energy can most easily flow. Then before you know it, you can't get out of those grooves. You might want to move in a new direction, but you can't! There's a real basis for that feeling of stuckness in your energy system.

We all have places where we're stuck in life, whether it's our bodies, habits, work, relationships, or parenting. If you think about it, stuckness is what most of us suffer from. It can look like not cleaning up your diet even though you really want to. Stuckness might be the creative project you've been talking about for two years but haven't started or the exercise regime you never follow through on. Stuckness is the intentions that never get acted upon and the recurring problems that you never take action to solve. It's the job or relationship you've been wanting to leave for ten years. It's any change that you've been too afraid to make. Or it could just be a feeling of stagnation in your body or your life that you can't seem to shake. If you feel flat most of the time instead of excited and energized, then you need to take a look at what's going on in your knees.

The energetic state of stuckness generates all kinds of feelings: frustration, anger, blame, victimhood, helplessness, sadness. So much of these feelings come from the inability to flow in a different or more effective way. By taking action to get out of the places where we've been stuck, there's a lot we can do to manage our emotional bodies and raise our voltages.

I invite you to take an inventory of where you feel stuck. Take a moment to breathe, center, and ground and think about the places in your life where you've been stalled, where you're in a state of inaction, or where you haven't been able to move forward. Keep those things in mind as you move through this chapter, and add to the list as you become aware of things you might not have realized before.

Now look beyond where you've been stuck. On the other side of stuckness is always liberation. It's the freedom to follow our natural inclinations, to allow our magnetic sense to guide us in life, to be moved into new and exciting directions. Turn your awareness to how nature is trying to move you. Where does your body want to go? What would you do if there was absolutely nothing blocking you? Tuning in to our internal guidance system is what clearing the knees is all about. Learning how to feel when it's time to go. Feeling when you want to do one thing and you don't want to do something else. Giving yourself permission to follow your natural inclinations and to speak your truth about it. That's not something we have to actively *try* to do—it comes naturally when we've cleared the noise and static that's getting in the way.

I love what Henry David Thoreau says: "I believe that there is a subtle magnetism in Nature, which, if we unconsciously yield to it, will direct us aright." To follow that magnetism—which is to say, to follow the inner pull of the soul's path and purpose—is our birthright. We know what this is, we feel it, it's obvious to us. Just like migrating birds and pollinating bees and other animals work with magnetic lines and energy, so do we. There are countless miraculous ways that your body uses its magnetic sense to guide its own growth and healing. We are a part of nature, and as such, it is healthy and instinctive for us to follow the flow of nature that tells us where to go and how to grow.

RIGHT KNEE: OBSTACLES MOVING FORWARD

The results of clearing up the energy in the knees can be dramatic. That is especially true of the right knee, where we hold the record of challenges or obstacles moving forward. There's almost a sense of water bursting through a dam as old blockages clear up and the energy starts flowing again.

When the right knee is blocked, it's typically a sign of self-sabotage, blocked action or stifled movement, undermining ourselves, or allowing ourselves to be undermined by others. There are all kinds of obstacles found here. Sometimes they come from outside: an unsupportive partner or helicopter parent, a mountain of student loan debt, the golden handcuffs of a high-paying but unfulfilling job. But just as often, they're internal: a story of unworthiness, a fear of failure, a fear of success, procrastination.

I once worked on a woman whose right knee was incredibly jammed up. She had been repeatedly blocked from her natural inclinations as a child, and later in life, she filled that role with her own self-sabotage when her parents were no longer there to do it for her. Tuning that knee took a long time, as it was jam-packed with story after story of her not being free. I was tuning and tuning and tuning her knee for what felt like hours, and finally, the energy started to clear and cohere. By the time we were done, it sounded clear as a bell. The next day, I received an email from her brimming with excitement over all the things she'd gotten done in the previous twenty-four hours. She finally made headway on a couple of work projects that had been stalling, she cleaned her kitchen, and she checked a few big items off her to-do list. She was finally able to break through all these little places in her life where she'd been backlogged. As soon as that energy went into flow, she could get out of her own way and get shit done. She moved through all her tasks effortlessly, with a sense of ease and enjoyment.

Countless times, I have seen incredible things happen to people when they unblock the right knee. Without any forcing or effort, they seamlessly move forward with tasks that have previously stymied them. Productivity increases in spades. It's as if your inner traffic lights have turned from red to green. When the right knee clears up, you have the energy to clean the whole house! There's a renewed capacity for swift and effective motion.

I once worked on a man in his early twenties who had been put on Ritalin at age nine. He had been told that he was hyperactive, that he was too lively. Adults shamed him over and over again for expressing his true self—the curious and lively child who wanted to go outside and not sit in a boring classroom under fluorescent lights. And so he had become terrified of the anticipated judgment and punishment that he would suffer if he acted as nature wanted him to. He had such a massive and charged block on the right side of his knee that the 528 Hz fork that I was using "blew"—it lost its structural integrity and became essentially useless. After the session, he said that he didn't realize just how much the fear of what other people thought had been holding him back. He later reported a surprising ease around feeling freer to do what he felt like doing without the voices of other people's judgment in his head.

For many people, the right knee keeps the score of other people's energy coming in and preventing us from following our natural inclinations. Another man, a longtime client of mine, first came to see me with right knee and hip pain. I remember when I was first working on his right knee and I hit the area in his field correlating roughly with the age of eighteen, the fork got really stuck. The resistance was so thick that moving the fork suddenly felt like pulling taffy. I asked him if anything had happened at that age.

"I really wanted to go to Harvard, and my parents wanted me to go to Yale," he said with a tone of regret in his voice. "That was the tradition in our family. My dad and his dad went to Yale. It was what they always wanted for me."

The pressure from his father was very intense, and he ended up going to Yale. His natural inclination was to go one way, but there were very powerful forces outside of him pushing him to go another way. While intellectually he had moved on from that experience, his body held the record of that blockage and all the disappointment, regret, and anger that came with it. What he was able to see clearly after the session was just how much it had impacted his ability to follow his natural impulses in other areas of his adult life.

As the oldest child in a large family, he had repeatedly been enlisted in helping take care of his younger siblings and also doing what his parents had wanted. He realized he was still living that way as an adult and that it had been impacting his health. The energetic pattern had destabilized the knee, resulting in right hip pain (which also was correlating to his overdoing for others, as we'll see in the next chapter). As you might imagine, in the light of this observation, he started choosing his actions more consciously rather than defaulting into accommodator mode.

Here's another example of an external blockage that became an inner obstacle to moving forward. One of my clients is a charming and talented young man who could have been a professional, number-one snowboarder. This guy was a total rock star: He was handsome, funny, and charismatic. He had all the drive and the talent in the world. He'd spent his entire childhood dreaming of becoming a pro snowboarder. There was nothing he loved more than being up on the mountain, crushing some fresh powder. But in his teens, at the time when he really needed to be supported in being at the mountain as much as possible, his parents weren't in a position to swing it. They didn't live near any ski areas, and they couldn't afford to get him to the mountains as much as he needed to continue his training. His deepest dream became something that he was never able to live out. On an energetic level, he got stuck there and never really grew up. The energy of that insurmountable obstacle became frozen in his field, and it kept him from moving on and pursuing new dreams. Losing that dream was a real trauma that created an experience of soul loss. When I worked on him, this energy showed up very prominently in both of his knees. In the right knee, the unresolved emotions stemming from that trauma showed up as an obstacle blocking him from taking action to materialize new dreams.

The tracks laid down in our early years become the path of our lives. All these examples are classic cases of an external blockage creating a pattern of self-sabotage: First, we're blocked by other people's energies, and then we start to block ourselves. Right-knee resistance can almost always be traced back to some external authority blocking your actions or self-expression when you were growing up. If you were constantly being told no, then when those characters go away, you start to do it to yourself. Even if nobody is there to say no to you anymore, you start to negate yourself because it's a familiar pattern. You repeat this story of *Something's going to come in and block me. Something is always going to undermine me. I might as well beat them to the punch.* That's the programming of your nervous system! These are the tracks that you'll find yourself stuck in.

It really doesn't matter what kind of parents you had. Through the process of domestication, we are all blocked to some degree or another from many of the natural urges that we have to express ourselves. As children, we learn to sit still, be quiet, stay in line, behave ourselves. If we've been constrained in this way in our upbringing, then we will continue to limit ourselves and put boundaries on our own movement and expression. We'll engage in self-sabotage because that's what we've been taught to do.

I was fortunate to be given an advantage in this department because of the way I was raised. I grew up in a family as the youngest of six kids. All my siblings were between six and twelve years older than I was, so by the time I came along, my parents were tired and pretty much ready to retire. They'd also learned a thing or two about parenting by the sixth time around. I was always told, "You go ahead and do what you feel like, Eileen." I had permission to follow my own internal referencing and do what felt right to me. Very few people are granted that kind of freedom. Having that as a child allowed me to feel comfortable taking risks to move forward with my internal nudgings. I had my parents' blessing to follow my own inclinations, so it was natural for me to do that later in life—the tracks had already been laid.

LEFT KNEE: ATTACHMENT AND RELEASE

A blockage in the right knee often has some connection to a blockage in the left. In the left knee, we hold on to old "stuff" from the past that no longer makes sense for us in our current lives. It could be anything that we feel ready to let go of—a marriage, an extra twenty pounds, a pile of junk in the garage—but for whatever reason, we can't bring ourselves to do it.

There's a lot of agonizing here about what to do next. I call it the knee of *Should I stay or should I go?* When this knee is clear and coherent, we know exactly when it's time to leave a relationship, a job, or a city. We're able to recognize when a substance, habit, or belief is no longer serving us, and we can take appropriate action to disengage from it. When it's not, we find ourselves engaged in an internal struggle about whether or not to leave.

It's related to the left-foot imbalance of being mired in a toxic situation that we feel powerless to change. The left foot, however, is largely unconscious. There's a sense of resignation and victimization that says, "Well, I guess this is just the way things are," which leads to a sense of disconnection and disassociation. But in the knee, there's a very conscious inner conflict about whether to try to change the situation. We spend a tremendous amount of energy going back and forth about it.

The left knee holds the devil you know. It's the relationships and attachments in our lives that we know aren't good for us but we can't seem to quit. So why do we stay? What it really comes down to is the ability to recognize when we've had enough and to trust that it's safe to let go. People who stay too long in jobs or relationships, or who struggle with addictions and dependencies, tend to have a hard time recognizing *satiation*. If you can't recognize when you've had your fill, it makes it difficult to say, "No, thank you," and walk away.

The healthy tonal expression of the left knee is this basic rhythm of getting your fill and moving on to the next thing. It's the ability to say, "Now I've had enough of that job, and it's time for me to find another job." The energy of the left knee then syncs up with the right knee to give you the force to actually go out and find that new job without blocking yourself with a bunch of excuses and stories about why you can't.

Left-knee imbalances are always issues of attachment and release. Think about it: if you weren't attached to the way things are, you wouldn't be stuck. This pattern often goes all the way back to our earliest attachment in life: the bond between mother and child. If you didn't bond well with your mom, whether because you didn't get enough skin-to-skin contact, or there was postpartum mental illness, or the environment was chaotic, you can end up with a lot of energy stuck here. Without an internal reference point for the feeling of satiation, of having your needs met, you'll find yourself in a continual state of frustrated desire and comfort seeking.

While the "stuff" we're attached to is often jobs and relationships that have run their course, it can be as deep as our energenetic patterning, the tone or rhythm of the song of our DNA. We can inherit a pattern of stress, of suppression, of sadness from our parents and our parents' parents that becomes an unhealthy attachment. I worked on a woman a few years ago, and it was evident in her left knee that she had inherited a chaotic, stressed-out frequency from her father, who was an alcoholic and whose own father was also an alcoholic. Her mother's energy, on the other hand, was sad and wiped out, with a sense of hopelessness and resignation. As a result, this woman had two powerful streams in her energy system with very distinct frequencies. She would wake up one day feeling depressed, and then the next day, she'd be stressed and agitated. She was constantly oscillating back and forth between these two emotional patterns, and no matter how much she tried, she couldn't seem to break out of them. What she thought was coming from herself was a case of energenetic patterns moving through time and space in her DNA as part of a process that had been going on long before her. Part of the work of getting her out of that pattern was releasing her attachment to it, which we did by tuning the field of the left knee.

When we don't extract ourselves from unhealthy situations of our own volition, life has a way of doing it for us—often in a way that's much more painful. That's when we get the "spiritual two-by-four." Life gives us all these gentle nudges that it's time to move along, starting with these little whispers telling us that we need to grow and embrace change. But if we're not paying attention, the two-by-four hits: the car accident, the firing, the court order. If you miss the cues because you haven't been listening, the decision gets made for you. Pretty much everyone I have ever worked with who suffered a serious accident or diagnosis answers yes to the following two questions: Were you stressed before this happened? Did it end up working out for the best? Life will find a way to put you on your path, even if it has to almost kill you to do it.

When the left knee is clear, we're less likely to get to that point because we've cleared the static enough to be able to hear the subtler nudges. Clarifying the left knee helps our inner knowing to arise. One thing that can help facilitate that process, when you're not sure which way to go, is to try directing your awareness into your gut and asking what you should do. Culturally, we tend to be given two choices: Go with your head or go with your heart, with your logic or your emotions. But there's a third option that's often left out, and that's your gut. Your gut tends to know where you need to go. I personally am a bigger fan of the gut than the head or heart when it comes to decision-making. While your head (intellect) is often stuck in the past and anticipated future, and your heart (emotions) are not always a reliable guide to what's really going on, your gut is comprised of a whole council of intelligent organs. Your liver is a brilliant commander of countless bodily systems and functions. Your spleen, pancreas, adrenals, stomach, and gallbladder . . . there's a tremendous amount of wisdom here. I mean, even your small intestine looks like your brain! We'll talk about this in detail in the solar plexus chapter, but for now, try connecting to an awareness of the center of your body and seeing what kind of inner knowing arises.

FINDING FREEDOM IN THE NOW

Sometimes I will encounter a stream of energy sort of circling from the fronts of the knees to about six or eight inches above them. I discovered that this is often an indication of what I call *greener pasture thinking*. It's a distinct energetic structure that's created when we habitually project ourselves into an imagined future where we'll be happy or free. *When I pay off my debt . . . When I lose the weight . . . When I have more energy . . . When I can finally leave my job . . .* It's the deferment of freedom, wholeness, and the ability to rest in contentment to some point on the horizon.

Point-on-the-horizon thinking is the opposite of living freely in the moment. When you feel that who you are and what you have at this moment is insufficient, then you're not free to be happy or complete or joyful right now. This is backward thinking! We are already whole. We're exactly where we need to be in this moment. The more we can sink into that feeling—nowhere to go, nothing to do, no ax to grind, no agenda to push, nothing to fix—the more we can live in a state of contentment.

When happiness is a can that's always being kicked down the road, the happy moment never comes. Meanwhile, you're surrounded by all the gifts and beauty and abundance of creation. There are miracles everywhere, but you're not letting them in.

There's a cartoon I love that perfectly captures this. It shows a guy and his dog sitting and watching a sunset. The dog has a thought bubble over his head with just a heart in it, while the guy has this whole cloud of thoughts hanging over him. The dog is in the moment, loving the fact that he gets to sit there watching this sunset. But the owner isn't able to enjoy that simple bliss because he's so caught up in the shit we've all got—all the mind viruses and stories and buggy programming. But what we all really want is to be in that dog's state: *Here I am, enjoying life. All is well, and I'm grateful.* How often do we feel this way?

This is the freedom we're looking for, and it only exists in the present moment. There's nowhere else to find it. The present moment is fluid and flowing. When you're fully in it, life becomes a dance. When you're out dancing and having a good time, you're not thinking, *Five steps from now, I'm going to be over there lifting my arms this way.* You're not waiting to enjoy the dance until your favorite song comes on. But that's what we do! We're not really in the present moment, which means that we're not moving freely. If you think of life as a dance, you can learn some of the steps, but ultimately, you just have to get on the floor and start moving your body. You just have to dive into the flow of your own being and everything around you. You have to trust the process of surrendering to your magnetic sense and allowing it to guide you.

SPONTANEOUS APPROPRIATE ACTION

Regardless of what's going on around us, we can to a large degree choose to breathe and center and be present right here and then allow spontaneous action to arise from that. Return to the flow of the moment by noticing what you are being nudged toward, what feels like it's ready to float downstream away from you. Be curious about your internal nudges, your inclinations, the things that spark inspiration and joy, and the emotions that come up when you start to follow them. (Hint: Guilt is a big one.)

The thing about spontaneous appropriate action and freedom in the feet and knees is that it's actually really easy. It's not a struggle. It's really just flow! The same way that water flows downriver or electricity flows along a current, we are meant to flow through our lives.

Moving through life in this way is like being a bird of prey gliding in the air. A hawk circling through the sky is so effortless and powerful at the same time. That's what flow feels like to me. It's a state of gliding through my day with a balance of strength and lightness. The trick to moving from our lives in this way, I believe, is simply to do more of what you enjoy doing. Catch the updrafts! Choose *ahh* over *uggh*. It's the feeling of *Ah, I'm free to do as I like. I can go this way instead of that way.* We become free when we allow ourselves to move and be moved, free to enjoy the moments of our lives as they unfold.

Freedom is always available. It doesn't come from anything external. You don't get freedom from something good happening or something bad going away. The *feeling* of freedom is primary; it comes first. If you want more freedom in your life, start embodying freedom right now. We're all actors and actresses. We can conjure up this feeling of freedom in our beings. Take five minutes to do that by taking a breath, centering your energy, and then asking yourself, *What does it mean for me to be free? What does that look like? How would I feel if suddenly everything I've been bound by all just fell away?* Experience that feeling of the debt, the self-doubt, the judgment, the obligations just falling away and floating downstream. Don't worry if it doesn't feel natural at first. Just allow yourself to be an actor, to conjure up the feeling of freedom, and to carry that with you into this moment and the next.

Emotional conjuring is a handy little exercise that you can practice with any feeling that you want to embody in your life. Approach it as a character study! Use your powers of imagination to call forth the thing you want to feel, and watch as it eventually becomes a familiar part of your being.

10

ROOT: Being and Doing

In the chakra system, our first energy center—the root, located at the base of the pelvis—deals with security and stability, livelihood and home, and our ability to take care of our basic survival needs. The color of the root chakra is red, the vowel sound is "uuhh," and the seed syllable is "LAM." In the biofield anatomy, the root also relates to our ability to take constructive action in our lives. It speaks to the connection between what we think and what we do. The energy that gets stuck here contains a record of disrupted doing and disrupted action. What I often see here is a kind of torque motion—a twisting, rotational force between overdoing and overthinking on the right side and frustrated non-doing on the left.

A healthy root chakra serves the function of being the overall battery meter for the system. It powers and supports everything sitting above it. If you think of your energy system in terms of the pyramid of Maslow's hierarchy of needs—which starts with survival needs and reaches all the way up to self-actualization—the foundation of the pyramid is the root base. If the root is solid, if you're centered and aligned in your actions, if you feel safe, you have a home, your basic needs are met, then you can work with all the energy centers that come above it. I've found that if people are going through a remodel and their homes are in chaos, their root chakras get all whacked out from it, and everything in their lives suffers as a consequence. If you're not taking care of the foundational issues housed here, if you're not storing energy properly at the base of your being, then you're going to be struggling at every level.

As the overall battery meter, the root determines how we're allocating our energetic resources. How much of your energy is being directed to your thinking mind? How much is going to your busyness and over-doing? How much is going toward spinning your wheels over *not* doing something? When the root energy is healthy and flowing, we know how to expend our energies. We know whether to take the elevator or the stairs. We understand our energies as a currency, and we're mindful about our deposits and withdrawals. If your root is healthy and strong, you will be energized and well rested. You don't have that constant background noise of tiredness and drag. You're conservative with your energy and judicious with how you spend it.

One of my Biofield Tuning instructors, Lori Rhoades, told us a great story about how she was driving home from the mall one day, put her hand in her purse, and realized her phone was not there. She immediately went into a panic and started expending lots of energy in a highly charged stress response. Then she realized, "I might as well have been driving down the highway and throwing twenty-dollar bills out the window." She reined herself in, took some deep breaths, and told herself that she was going to find it. She went back to the shopping center and discovered that it was waiting for her at a store she had been in. Lori made a conscious choice to not spend her energetic currency foolishly (nothing will drain your battery faster than panic!) by using her mind and her breath firmly and directively.

Working with the energy of the root helps us find coherence around our balance of being versus doing. We learn to follow our own natural rhythms of where our energies want to go, knowing when it's time to go to bed, take a day of rest, eat more fruit, or whatever else we might need to do (or *not* do) to manage our energy levels.

In our physical anatomy, the root relates to the pelvis, tailbone, and reproductive organs. In some models, the adrenals are part of the endocrine system associated with the root. While I tend to place them in the solar plexus where they are physically located, I do often hear adrenal-related alarm bells going off in this area. In my estimation, it has to do with the survival and safety concerns that are housed here. Was home a safe place when you were a child? Were there people yelling? Was your mom stressed out from trying to work full-time and take care of everyone? When we hit early childhood on the right side of the root, there's often a sense of hypervigilance and needing to protect ourselves. This is a very core adrenal activity. It's in these early years that we made the decision whether the world is a safe place or an unsafe place.

Many systems also connect the root chakra to the immune system, which makes sense considering that immunity is directly related to our internal batteries. The more voltage we have, the more power in our immune systems. The higher our batteries, the more of an army we've got. When the battery gets low, morale gets low. We lose some of our troops. The body has to decide how and where to allocate resources, and when that happens, it's going to take energy away from one area to send it to another. That's how we become susceptible to disease.

In the biofield anatomy, the left side of the root speaks to a sense of *frustrated non-doing:* it's the things we want to do, be, or have but that we are not currently doing, being, or having. There's a sense of spinning our wheels, often stemming from an old pattern of frustration over unmet needs. The field to the right of the root speaks to being busy, but not necessarily with the things we'd like to be doing. Here we find the energy of overthinking and guilt-driven overdoing; overworking, over-busyness, overachieving and over-approval-seeking. The "back" of the root chakra, which descends from the tailbone straight down the legs, relates to our physical homes and the degree of noise or harmony in our houses, cars, offices, desks, or studios. The essential vibrations of our immediate environment, whether that's cluttered and chaotic or clear and calming, show up here. Here, I also find those survival fears related to our early home lives and worries about making a living and being able to pay our rents or mortgages.

There is a kind of placidness in a healthy and balanced root chakra, like a deep-keeled boat. We trust ourselves and the universe, knowing that we're safe and our needs will be provided for. We're connected to the earth and drawing that nourishing energy up into our systems. We're able to rest in a relaxed, aware presence bolstered by a deep sense of security in ourselves and our beings.

RIGHT SIDE: OVERTHINKING AND OVERDOING

In the early days of Biofield Tuning, I was consistently finding that most people were running the majority of their energies off their right hips. It baffled me. What I came to discover here over time was one of the most profound and universal imbalances in the field.

I mentioned in Part I that there is a core structure in the biofield anatomy, located around fourteen to eighteen inches off the right side of the right hip. It feels almost like the wheel of a wheelchair spinning parallel to the body. I call it the *busy mind wheel*. This is something I find in almost everyone, and it shows up as a deep structural imbalance in the energy body. It's the energetic imprint of a mind that runs off like a wild horse into to-do lists, "Gotta get it done," worrying about the future, concerns about what other people think, guilt, self-criticism. And if we move in along that same line of energy to roughly eight to ten inches from the body, we find the *busy body wheel* of constant work, motion, and activity.

Because of this dual structure, I call the right hip *the hip of chronic overdoing*. People who are chronically busy will often end up with right hip issues like arthritis and sciatica. I have seen a ton of clients with right hip replacements and very few with left hip replacements. There is also a spinning wheel structure that exists off the left hip (and we'll talk about that in a moment), but it tends to be less pronounced.

When your mind is racing, it feels like it's happening in your brain, but on an energetic level, it's also happening here off the right hip. We redirect and drain a huge amount of energy off our bodies in this pattern. This is energy that wants to be in the body in circulation! But instead, it's siphoned out into this overly yang energy of *I gotta stay busy, I gotta make money, I gotta be productive, I gotta run this side hustle, I gotta keep it all together.* This has become such a "normal" way of being in our modern lives that we've lost sight of just how phenomenally dysfunctional it is. Living in a state of overdoing and overthinking is *wildly* out of balance. It's very linear and goal oriented. It's a mind that doesn't shut up and a body that can't sit still. I see this imbalance to some degree in nearly everyone.

This energy vortex off the right side of the root chakra traps earth energy, or what we might think of as kundalini, and keeps it from rising up and ascending through the rest of the body. Instead of traveling up the central channel the way it naturally wants to, the energy is getting diverted and going into a spin. This is where the greatest amount of our potential gets diverted. When I do group sessions, it shows up as a collective frenzy of busyness, overworking, productivity obsession, go-go-go, do-do-do, and chronic stress that leads to burnout.

I attribute the universality of this pattern to a deep collective hyperactivity in our culture. While most energetic imbalances are rooted in the individual and familial, cultural and societal imbalances make their mark on us, too. We exist in the spaces between one another, in the collective electromagnetic field, and we're far more influenced by the larger environment than we tend to think. Whenever I'm in Canada, I always notice how different the people are there, even though they're located right next to us geographically and our cultures look outwardly quite similar. But the energy of Canadians is so different from that of Americans! The morphic field of Canada informs the humans who inhabit that environment and influences them in profound ways, and the right-hip wheel is *much* less pronounced in Canadians than it is in Americans. The frequency of capitalist-driven hyperproductivity exists around the world, but it is much more apparent in the fields of folks living in the United States.

The stress of being a human in modern culture puts us at a pace that's overly yang, high octane and cranked up, like we've had too much caffeine. Scientists have even found that the human heartbeat, instead of being around sixty beats per minute, has risen to roughly eighty beats per minute. This is not a natural state of being! It's a blind obedience to the hustle that has separated us from our natural flow and expression. A 2019 headline in *The Atlantic* summed it up well: "The Religion of Workism Is Making Americans Miserable."

We see people like Elon Musk, who works forty hours a week in one of his companies and forty hours a week in another, and that's held up as our standard. Or former Yahoo! CEO Marissa Mayer, who says that anyone can manage a 130-hour workweek "if you're strategic about . . . how often you go to the bathroom." This is a universal, but particularly American, template. It's a mold that needs to be broken.

We need to start to understand busyness as a profound energetic imbalance. It is not a natural state of being. I repeat: *Busyness is not a natural state of being!* Habitual overworking, overachieving, overscheduling, over-pleasing and over-approval-seeking is not conducive to health, happiness, or performance in the long run. It leads to stress, burnout, and exhaustion, and it takes an enormous amount of energy away from the vital functions of the body.

OVERCOMING THE ADDICTION TO DOING

At its extreme, overworking and over-busyness is an addiction, and it's one of the most difficult addictions to overcome. Why? Because it looks so good! You're getting things done. You're impressing others, or at least keeping up with them. It's also handy because you don't even need any substance. You don't have to have wine or chocolate in the house. There's no end to ways that you can go off the rails with busyness.

When you're so busy doing for everyone else, you're not doing the things that matter. You're not getting to your art or your music or your poetry. Your walks in nature. Even your lunch with your girlfriends. We get into this martyr drudgery, the drone of "must get everything done." We don't ask for help. What I call the *doing virus* has this isolating effect that makes it difficult for us to connect and receive. What happens most of the time is that we run around in circles with all kinds of busywork but don't get the rubber on the road with the things that are truly meaningful to us.

Like any other addiction, it is a way that we numb and dissociate from our bodies and our emotions. Being in constant motion is a way to avoid our feelings, particularly sadness. Some people use alcohol, some people use food, but a lot of people in our culture use motion. We keep going so that our emotions never have a chance to settle. As long as you're listening to the voice in your head and manically trying to make your way through your bottomless to-do list, you don't have to listen to the sound of your own pain. A hyperactive mental body overrides the emotional body. This is a huge part of why people spin out in their heads. Many bodyworkers, myself included, have noted a correlation between the right hip and the left shoulder. Right hip imbalances of overthinking and overdoing are often the counterpoint to the issues on the left side of the heart chakra, which holds unprocessed sadness, loss, and grief.

When you start to quiet the mind and slow the busyness down, the feelings you've been avoiding *will* come up. That's a good thing, because those emotions are stuck energy that's creating resistance and drag in your field, your mind, and your life. It can be uncomfortable, and it does take a little time to settle back to neutral. But as you move through your own emotional backlog, you liberate a huge amount of your own potential. You free up energy to be expressed in creative and fun and pleasurable ways. You start to return to the juiciness and magic and depth of the moment that you were missing out on when you had the right side of your field all scrunched up in a bunch.

BECOMING ALPHA OVER YOUR THOUGHTS

A busy body is often driven by a busy mind, so the mind is the place to begin dismantling the doing virus and getting our freedom back.

I often liken the thinking mind to having a bad dog (or multiple bad dogs!) in our heads that doesn't sit, stay, or stop barking. It doesn't come when we say, "Come." It eats the garbage. It's completely undisciplined. But we're not completely powerless over it. We have to make the decision to find the part of us that can discipline that dog and go ahead and discipline it! This is a process that takes time, but there are some tools and approaches that can help. We have to do it with love, like we'd discipline our toddler. It took thirteen years before I didn't have to remind my kids every day to brush their teeth, but then finally, they did it on their own. That's the way the thinking mind is! It takes years of constant reminders and discipline to quiet it down.

Just because you and just about everyone you know has a pack of wild dogs living in their heads doesn't mean that it's appropriate or necessary. There is a part of you that is not your thoughts that has to be alpha, that has to be in control of those dogs. It's an ongoing process, but by using tools like sound to rebalance the energy of our root center and by *choosing* to be in control of our minds, we can begin to take charge of our thoughts.

I used to have mastiffs—a 180-pound female English mastiff and then a 220-pound male. They're massive dogs. If you have a dog that big, you have to be in charge. You have to be alpha. If you're not commanding, dogs like that just don't pay attention, but if you are going to be a good big dog owner, you can't take no for an answer! That's the kind of discipline—the "big dog voice"—that's required to deal with our unruly minds. Your mind is going to take you down if you don't take some control. You have to find the part of you that is not your thinking mind that will not tolerate having a pack of bad dogs in your head.

Having a mastiff taught me a lot about that kind of commanding nature that we have and that we need to get into at times. We have to figure out a way to get in touch with effective inner discipline. When I'm commanding my dog, I'm not being aggressive or mean to him. I'm not being cruel or unkind. I'm just using the appropriate amount of firmness to get the job done. It's more about being strong. It's not the voice of your inner critic—it comes from this deeper place inside that's responsible for keeping your organism healthy and being true to yourself.

I invite you to be willing to get over the belief that you don't have control over what is going on in your own head. If you don't have control over your thoughts, who does? Are the thoughts running themselves? Take responsibility for that mind of yours, grab the reins, and start to experiment exercising a firm authority over your runaway, unproductive thought loops.

Keep in mind uncontrollable thinking is usually an indication that you are trying to think your emotions, rather than actually feel them! We get stuck in loops of mental attack and defense when we are trying to avoid uncomfortable feelings like shame. Drop out of your head and into your body, and allow yourself to really feel what is going on. Allow those feelings to rise and crest and then they will pass, I promise! When they have passed, you will find it is easier for your mind to settle.

LEFT SIDE: FRUSTRATED NON-DOING

The overdoing imbalance on the right side of the root chakra inevitably hurtles us back over to the left side: inertia, and what I've come to see as *frustrated non-doing*. It holds feelings of frustration over needs that aren't being met, the things we really want to be doing but don't have the time or energy for, and the places in our lives where we can't seem to get the rubber on the road. When we're running around with all kinds of busy-work, we're often not getting to the things that are actually anything meaningful, productive, or creatively fulfilling for us, and we feel frustrated as a result.

Whatever thoughts and desires you're turning around in your head but not turning into concrete steps—whether it's a dietary change or a new creative project—the accumulation of that unexpressed energy is going to pool around the left hip. I sometimes think of it as the "hip of quiet desperation," as it contains such a great deal of unrealized potential—as well as unfulfilled emotional needs that we have denied and disconnected from. The energy that gets trapped here is pure light, pure potential, that's been frustrated, scattered, given away, and stuck. It's very connected to the stuckness found in the knees and feet.

The question to ask yourself here is, *Where in your life are you not getting the rubber on the road?* Maybe you want a new car or job and you can't seem to save the money. Or you want to exercise and eat better, but you can't seem to take the first steps. You want to leave your corporate job, but you're afraid to take the risk to launch your own venture. These are experiences of frustrated non-doing. Consciously, you want it, but something in the subconscious mind is blocking or arresting it. There's a tension that comes from being inwardly divided, but it's also a divide between you and your manifesting ability and creative power.

Frustration is the natural result when we're not acting in alignment with our needs and desires. This comes up a lot when we're out of alignment between what we think we want and the subconscious habits we're acting out. So what's the deal? Why can't we just bring ourselves to *do* the thing we so desperately want to do? What's often happening here is that we're re-creating and reenacting a pattern of frustration over unmet needs that's been familiar since early childhood. If your basic needs weren't being met early in life—and especially if you didn't feel safe or secure in your home—it becomes extremely difficult to switch gears and become proactive in attending to your own needs as an adult. You have to learn to become your own parent and nurture yourself.

A lot of people who try to make lifestyle changes end up stuck in that left hip. I worked with a woman once who had been trying to lose weight for years. She had a huge amount of frustration around her desire to take care of her health on the one hand and her seeming inability to stop eating too many empty calories on the other. What we found was that she had certain circumstances in her childhood that led to her not feeling safe, and that comforting herself with carbohydrates was a coping strategy she'd taken on as a teenager to suppress that feeling of being unsafe. It became a kind of ritual and comfort. The forks also revealed that she had a lot of stagnation and sense of emptiness in her solar plexus. By eating, she was bringing movement and activity into this area, bringing a temporary sense of warmth and comfort to her inner void. Overeating was actually serving her! That's why it was so hard to give up. It made her feel safe and cared for. And because the underlying feeling of a lack of safety had not been resolved, she kept on reaching for the coping mechanism that was making her feel better. With any of our compulsions, addictions, or any behaviors that we are in inner conflict around, we always need to ask ourselves, *How am I using this to feel safe?*

When you're in that state of frustrated, spinning energy, when you're struggling to align your needs and desires with your actions, it's helpful to step back into the state of mind known as *the witness*. Look at yourself from a perspective beyond yourself and acknowledge that you've got your biofield all in a bunch! You're clamped down around your left hip, running this old story of frustration that's been going for God knows how many years. Can you step back and let go of it and settle into neutral?

Notice when you're spinning out in frustration and come back to what's happening in your body in the here and now.

FINDING RIGHT LIVELIHOOD

Right smack in the center of the root chakra, between guilt-driven over-doing and frustrated non-doing, we discover what the Buddhists call *right livelihood*. Right being. Right doing. Right action. If you're aligned in your feet and knees and you have a strong root to support you, then you're doing your thing. You're going with the flow. You're a balanced human being, whatever that looks like for you. By bringing awareness to our patterns of chronic overdoing and frustrated non-doing, we can return the energy of the root to its rightful place—and to action that not only enlivens us but contributes positively to the collective.

Right livelihood means being engaged in actions that are true to our gifts. We are doing what we were built to do. We're experiencing genuine freedom and abundance through our actions. *That* is the idealized expression of the root chakra. We're centered and grounded, we're present, we're not in fear. We're not trying to be somewhere else or striving to fix anything. It's just a place of pure centered being, which supports our ability to move with the flow of life into the actions that are best suited for us. It's balancing our doing with our being in the way that best serves ourselves and others. I know that's an ideal, but I think it's important to hold and aim for ideals. (I call myself an unapologetic idealist, because someone has to be!)

Balancing doing and being means giving ourselves permission to pause all the frenzied activity and flow in a way that feels natural to us. Repeat after me: *I give myself permission to not run around like a crazy person.* I give you permission to take your time with what you need to do—not lollygagging but moving at the appropriate speed without fear of not getting everything done. We run around in circles with all kinds of busy-work. But it's important to question what you've really done at the end of the day and whether you've accomplished anything of value.

And more important, where are *you* in this equation of all these things you're running around and doing? Once we feel like we have permission to move from our centers in a state of flow, then we start to move toward the things that are appropriate for us at the pace that is most optimum. It can sound a little radical to have permission to do that rather than just marching forward and doing all the things our minds and our culture are telling us we have to do, but I'd like to invite you to really soak in the possibility of coming from a more deeply centered and easeful place in your everyday dealings with life. Aim to be like the bird of prey, gliding powerfully and effortlessly through your day.

Part of getting to a place of mental and emotional freedom is slowing down. Slowing down our brain waves, our heart rates, our monkey minds. Slow and steady is the way of health, happiness, and success in the long term. Invite spaciousness and pause and repose in your body and your mind and your day. When you're running a program of over-busyness, there's a tendency to constrict the chest and the diaphragm, to stop breathing and go into automatic-doing mode. That's when we need to connect to ground and discharge. Allow any excess energy to move through and out your feet. Trust that your body knows how to discern what's needed and what's not. You don't have to worry about making any conscious decisions about that. If you are overly fixated on the future, say, "I trust my future self to take care of that appropriately."

I am reminded of a woman at a class in Toronto who came in with her coffee on the last day of class and told us the story of what she was experiencing after having her right root worked on the day before. "I realized that I was centered in my body and just sort of flowing along," she said. "Usually, I feel like my thoughts and my mind are out in front of me, like I am always rushing to get here or there. But today, as I was heading to the coffee shop, I felt centered, present, in a true state of ease. It feels great!"

One of the core lessons of the root is that it's okay to rest. It's okay to take breaks. Remember that you're in this life for the long haul! You want to be the tortoise, not the hare. The hare is this energy of running around with busywork but not making meaningful progress in the direction of our creativity, our authenticity, our truth. The tortoise is slow, steady movement in the direction of our true needs and desires.

AVOIDING BURNOUT

I have always been a very hardworking person, but my lack of boundaries and inability to carve out time for self-care when I was younger led me to serious burnout not once but twice in my life. Between receiving tuning and learning boundaries and practicing some simple mind hacks that I will share here, I have been able to learn to practice *conservation of energy*. This practice has allowed me to spend the last five years teaching and traveling and growing a business virtually nonstop, without going into burnout or exhaustion. I call these *tubing* and *following updrafts*.

One great way to conserve energy is to refuse to rush and to diligently keep your inner speed akin to the experience of going inner tubing on a river. If you have ever gotten into an inner tube and floated down a river on a hot summer day, you understand what I mean—you are laid-back, just flowing along. Sometimes you hit some rapids and you go faster, but you are still in that laid-back, easy posture. When you are tubing, there is no urgency, no rushing, no struggling. It really is like being a tortoise.

And while I am keeping that inner speed nice and easygoing, I am also following updrafts, which means taking on whatever task feels easiest and has the greatest sense of "ahh!" around it (as opposed to "uggh"). Getting frothy when you are running around like a chicken with its head cut off, trying to do too much in too little time, or forcing ourselves to do something we really don't want to do are massive energy drains and, in many instances, not at all necessary but rather just happening by the force of habit. By tubing and updrafting, I can still get enormous amounts of things done. The trick to mastering this way of gliding through your day is trusting in yourself to get everything done that needs to be done! The key, again, is returning to center, to electromagnetic equilibrium. The more aligned in our centers we become, the more energy is flowing through our central axes.

I also like to practice regular, short (five minutes or less) micro-rests throughout my day. My favorite micro-rest is a simple meditation in which you imagine the torus shape of your energy field and feel into your central channel. The central channel is always open, but when you're getting all scrunched into overthinking and overdoing or frustration, that's when you can bring your awareness back into your toroidal electric body. Feel your central axis, and use your mind to bring yourself back into alignment. You can do this with your eyes open or closed, no matter where you are: Just take a minute to orient yourself and return back to your axis. Hold the space between heaven and earth, and just rest in that! That only takes a minute. Rein in your mind and energy, come to center and ground. Take some of those deep breaths into the belly and down into the earth. Look up at the sky and listen to the birds. Enter into an alpha brain wave state where your mind is at rest and you are simply listening to what is going on in the world around you. Rest in that for a moment, and then keep moving.

11

SACRAL: Reclaiming Pleasure, Worthiness, and Abundance

The sacral chakra is a bubbling cauldron of energy that houses our self-worth, sexuality, creativity, cash flow, and the ability to enjoy pleasure and intimacy—all things that most people in our culture don't have such a healthy relationship with! How many people do you know who are able to fully enjoy receiving money, intimacy, and pleasure without guilt? In my experience, it's very few.

Many people want to have the experience of being creatively juicy and sexy and abundant, and yet there are so many inner hurdles to getting to that place. The second energy center is jam-packed with so much "stuff" in just about everyone that it's almost ridiculous. It's really the messiest chakra on a collective level. In almost everyone I worked with in the early days of my practice, I found that the energy of the sacral center was spread like peanut butter across the field. There's a lot of scattered, stuck energy that inhibits flow across this region. On the right side of the chakra, we find guilt and shame, as well as the voice of the inner critic. On the left side lives frustration and disappointment; the scars of sexual transgressions, abortions, difficult births, and pregnancies; feeling unwanted or unloved; digestive issues; and struggles around receiving pleasure, intimacy, power, and money. To get back to the healthy frequency of the sacral, we can utilize the color orange, the vowel sound "oooo" and the seed syllable "VAM."

When we're in the sacral, we're getting into the emotions and mental programming that seem to most undermine people's health and well-being. In the physical anatomy, imbalance and interference signals here show up in lower GI disorders like IBS, SIBO, Crohn's, colitis, candida overgrowth, and gut microbial imbalances. I have identified a strong correlation of IBS with chronic and suppressed frustration, while Crohn's disease and colitis are almost always connected to a patterning of guilt, shame, and an overactive inner critic. Lower back pain often has to do with a strong suppression of any and all the emotions connected to this chakra. The sacral is also connected to prostate issues and anything to do with the uterus or other female reproductive organs.

Many spiritual traditions, especially in the East, had a strong reverence for this part of the body and the power it contains. The area just below the navel is often seen as the seat of consciousness. In Taoist alchemical texts, it's referred to as "the cauldron of desire," where our creative energy is stored. In Zen, it's the *hara*: the physical and spiritual center of the body. Students of Zen Buddhism are often instructed to train their attention on the *hara* as a technique for attaining control over their thoughts, emotions, and desires. It is literally the place from which we create life: the womb.

That's something that's been lost in our culture. This energy center has become very suppressed and diseased in the West—as evidenced in epidemic levels of digestive issues and lower GI disorders. Instead of the vibrant tone of aliveness that is the healthy expression here, what I hear much more often is a muffled under-the-rug tone that indicates a huge amount of energy below the surface that's being stifled and shut down. There's so much raw power here that we've been taught to be afraid of, and what I've seen is that nearly all of us have far more second chakra energy than we allow ourselves to experience.

A big part of that story is that religion has taken this fiery, primal creative force and put the face of the devil on it. As a result, there's an encultured tendency for people to dissociate and go numb in their sacral areas. When I guide students in taking their awareness through the chakras, I always observe how they struggle to keep their awareness in this part of the body. Many people can't even breathe into their bellies because they don't want to connect with all the guilt, shame, frustration, and disappointment that lives there. It's a wasps' nest of discomfort! Somewhere along the line, many people simply decide that they don't want to go there.

Just think about how we've been conditioned to look at this part of our bodies. All of us—but especially women—are taught from an early age to judge our bellies if we don't have the flat stomachs of models and athletes. It becomes the focus of our self-judgment and shaming. Instead of anchoring our consciousness in the belly with pleasure and enjoyment, there's a withdrawal and shaming. When we look at it from the outside with judgment and loathing and all kinds of stories, there's a rejection of this entire part of our beings that is the very center of creative power and inner knowing. We end up being *outside* of it instead of occupying it.

I'm calling for a reoccupation of the sacral chakra. We want to get back in there because it's where all the juiciness is. It's worth the discomfort of going into these places, breathing through them, and digesting them to get to that place of pleasure. Wading through the swamp of guilt and shame isn't easy, but the rewards are immense. Having a nice, clear second chakra opens up your power as a creator. It can take a bit of time and practice to wake up this part of the body, but I assure you that it can be done.

I also offer a warning: Working with this energy is incredibly potent. It gets a lot of deep hidden energies moving. Be gentle with yourself and really take some time in your own exploration of this part of your being. Sit with what comes up here, but don't get too bogged down in it. If you start experiencing fear, see if you can interpret that fear with a more positive spin. It's *exciting* to reclaim our right to pleasure, enjoyment, creativity, and resource flow! It's downright thrilling to embrace your worthiness to allow this energy to move freely through you. It puts you right at the front edge of your being, living an inspired, passionate life.

THE MYTH OF ORIGINAL SIN

The big signal jammer of the sacral chakra is the story of "I'm not good enough." *I'm not worthy of love. I don't deserve pleasure. I don't deserve the good things in life. I'm not worthy of being abundant. I'm not worthy of my own creative brilliance.* Where we have these beliefs, we hold our breaths, we block our energies, and very often our judgmental thoughts create static that generates a self-fulfilling prophecy. These beliefs are often so deeply programmed—stemming from forces that came before us and are much bigger than we are—and so habitual that we are largely unaware of their powerful influence over our lives.

Doing sacral work on groups and individuals, I've sometimes come across an interesting construct on the edge of the field, which I identified as the *veil of forgetting.* The tone feels like a layer of fog. What it tells me is that when we're born, we get this kind of amnesia. We forget who we are, and we forget our souls' missions. It's like we pass through a membrane that scrambles everything as we come into this dense, strange world. Then we have to go through our lives trying to remember our true identities. We forget that we are perfect and whole and complete—that we are the stuff of the stars—and as we are programmed and conditioned by our families and our culture, as we go through life's struggles and challenges, we come to identify with a self that's guilty and bad and wrong. We completely lose contact with the harmonic perfection of our souls.

When I first discovered the perfect harmony underneath the noise and static in everyone I worked on, it created a lot of cognitive dissonance for me. I was confused. As I tried to make sense of what I was encountering, I came to recognize my own belief that we are all guilty sinners who had fallen from grace. Like the first man and woman, Adam and Eve, we've been cast out of the garden. We are fundamentally flawed. We're all bad apples somehow. This was my subconscious belief—and I wasn't even raised in a religious home! I never went to church or Sunday school, but I had been inoculated with the virus of this belief in original sin.

And then here I was, seeing with my own eyes and hearing with my own ears something so different. I was experiencing these rainbow bodies of harmonic perfection—in everyone—and it didn't line up with what I had been programmed to believe about human nature.

My guess is that you hold this belief in some form, too, whether or not you were raised in a religious home. It's a nearly universal human myth that's almost impossible to avoid in modern culture. At some point in your life, you drank the Kool-Aid and came to believe on some level that you're a guilty sinner. And because of that, you've blocked yourself from greatness, from your innate brilliance, and from enjoying pleasure because you've been programmed with this dark triad of "guilty, bad, and wrong."

Ask yourself about your own relationship to the story of original sin. Was it something you were brought up with? Can you pinpoint a time in your childhood when you first started to feel "not good enough"? What are the experiences in your life today that tend to trigger these stories?

What happens energetically when you believe you're not worthy is that you block flow. Your nature is health and abundance, just like nature itself. Nature is riotously abundant. We're part of nature, and when you're in that flow, that is your experience of life. You have moments where you feel like you're just bursting into bloom and dripping with scented petals. We have those experiences because that's what we are, and yet there's this powerful subconscious programming that tells us we're not! Rather than being a part of nature's divine glory, we've been kicked out of Eden. We've fallen from grace. We did something bad, and we need to be punished. These stories are the kernel of almost every dysfunction in our lives. But they're just stories. It's noise in the signal that can be consciously removed.

When you start to think of yourself as nature, you start to think of yourself as *what you really are* beyond what you've been told, what we have been collectively programmed with. Think about the hardware you are composed of: You are made up of stardust and minerals and water and light. What's unworthy about that? You are stewarding a collection of molecules of creation; is there something unworthy about those molecules? If not, then why would the whole be lesser than the sum of its parts? As a part of nature, you are perfect, and to say anything other than that is simply untrue.

Take a big breath!

RIGHT SIDE: GUILT AND SHAME

The emotions of guilt and shame live on the right side of the sacral chakra. I have found these to be two of the most uncomfortable and disabling emotions that we can feel, because they are so deeply connected to this question of worthiness. They often run very subconsciously. We feel inadequate and bad about ourselves so regularly that we're not even aware that this has become our underlying emotional baseline.

What's the difference between the two? While guilt is best understood as "I did something bad," shame is the voice that tells us, "I *am* bad." That makes shame a bit heavier and harder to deal with. Shame, in my experience, is the single most uncomfortable emotion for people to feel. We run our mental bodies into overdrive as a way to avoid the overwhelming pain of feeling not good enough and not worthy of love and belonging.

In many cases, these emotions are related to sexual experiences—abortions, sexual assault, and childhood sexual abuse. I often find the area containing sexuality (and very often body shame along with it) to be like a snake's den of charged-up, uncomfortable energy. Among women who have been sexually abused as young girls, the field often reveals a loss of light and exuberance. There's this bright, shiny, happy starlight energy that's been dampened and downcast and made to feel ashamed.

Guilt and shame can originate in utero. This happens among children who were born out of wedlock or to mothers who, for whatever reason, felt shame around being pregnant. A pattern of guilt and shame can also originate in childhood when parents use these emotions to discipline and manipulate. It's around two years old that I often start hitting the tone of *no*, and consequently, the waveforms of guilt and shame begin to surface. This is when many children first start to experience punishment and reprimanding. *No, that's bad. No, you're being bad. No, don't do that. No, you're wrong.* Children are shamed for countless behaviors, including ones that are completely benign. I've seen time and again that they get shamed for just expressing their essential aliveness. We're shamed as a way to subdue our natural exuberance early in life. It's no wonder that we feel deadened as adults and dissociated from our creative life forces.

I frequently trace this pattern even further back. There's a huge amount of familial and ancestral influence in this chakra—meaning the patterns here don't even come from us! If you're American, there's a good chance that your ancestors experienced an extreme suppression of creative and sexual energy. We carry that distortion from the Puritans that came before us. We may also carry the distortion created by generations of female oppression. In the sacral chakra more than any other, we come preloaded with these knots that we have to untie to get to a place of liberation.

One of my students worked with a woman of Peruvian heritage who was a powerful intuitive and healer but had been afraid to share her gifts with others. There were significant imbalances on both sides of her sacral chakra stemming from her childhood and maternal lineage. It turned out that the women in her family were healers and medicine women, but many had repressed these gifts thanks to an inherited fear of persecution from the Catholic Church (as is common in many South American cultures). Through a series of sessions, they worked on releasing inherited fears stemming from her maternal grandmother and mother, as well as the stories that the client was telling herself about how claiming her feminine healing power would be going against God and Church. As she was able to release the ancestral patterning, she was able to step into her power as a healer.

Sound therapy or other forms of energy work can be hugely beneficial in depatterning these kinds of ancestral influences. There's also a simple, self-guided visualization that I like to use. First, just take a moment to breathe and ground your energy. Once you feel centered, close your eyes and visualize your second chakra as a glowing orange orb just below your navel. Imagine it as healthy, whole, vibrating, and aligned with its original blueprint. Shining strong, free from any guilt or blame or judgment or suppression. Then call to mind your mother and father and their relationship to their second chakras. Consider their relationship to money, creativity, and pleasure. Hold them in your vision, and then give them a bright, healthy, alive orange light shining below their navels. See their sacral chakras as healthy and whole, free from all the repression and suppression. Imagine them free from guilt and shame. Then do the same thing with all your ancestors, the ones you know as well as the ones you don't know. It may not be easy at first, but keep going. If all kinds of gunk comes up as you attempt to do this, that's okay. If you stay with it and trust that you will move through it, the waves will crest and then fall away.

No matter how bad these emotions might make you feel, remember that they're not inherently bad. Guilt and shame are uncomfortable, but they serve a purpose. Like the rumble strips on the side of the highway, they're there to help you stay in balance and to tell you when you've gotten off track. If you didn't feel any guilt or shame, you'd be a sociopath! The expression "Have you no shame?" speaks to the importance of feeling shame. Isn't the inability to feel shame and admit to wrong-doing the definition of a narcissist? A person who can't feel ashamed of bad behavior is not someone we want to be. Guilt and shame, when expressed in healthy ways, can help us to regulate our own behaviors and motivate us toward positive change where it's appropriate.

We want to be able to let the wave of the emotion wash through us, get the lesson, and then move on. What we *don't* want is to end up either avoiding these emotions or overindulging in them. As you go through your day, be aware of when you're indulging guilt and shame. Know when you're going into these heavy places. Use your mind to slide your energy back to center, and find something to be grateful for. And as always, breathe into the belly, center, and ground. Bring your energetic posture into neutrality when you're starting to tilt off. Know that you *can* command your photons and bring yourself into love and gratitude (unless, of course, what you really need to do in that moment is puddle).

We often seek to circumvent guilt and shame by projecting it onto others. I've seen many times that people will try to release these feelings of shame by going into blame and self-righteousness—both of which sit in the half-step zone between the solar plexus and sacral center, *above* guilt and shame. As long as you're in that place of thinking you're superior and making someone else the problem, you don't have to sink down into the discomfort of your own shame. But to actually heal, you will need to be willing to dive deep into your shame to release its accumulation in your system. (This is not a fun process, but it sure feels great on the other side!)

Note: I have observed that self-righteousness is a stealth enemy of peace of mind. Pay attention to when you are acting self-righteous about something, and notice how the energy arranges itself in your field when you are feeling that way. See if you can bring yourself back to center and take a deeper look at what is really going on.

TAMING THE INNER CRITIC

Guilt and shame give rise to judgment, and along with it, the construct of the inner critic. The inner critic is the single biggest thief of second chakra energy. It sits over on the right side of the lower belly and almost vampirically sucks away our creative forces. I see the chatter of the inner critic as parasitic thought forms that are feeding on our energies. It's a very dysfunctional dynamic that creates a lot of problems in a lot of people. To the extent that the inner critic is running the show, our digestion, joy, aliveness, and personal power are undermined.

Often, the inner critic takes the form of an inner perfectionist that never really lets you enjoy anything, because it should be better or different. *It's not good enough. I should be doing more. I could have done it better. Why can't I just be more like her/him/them?* The inner critic feeds the spinning wheel of busy mind and busy body off the right hip. Much of our relentless nonproductive overthinking and overdoing is driven by the voice, sitting in the field directly above that spinning wheel, that is constantly reminding us how we're falling short.

If you listen closely to your inner critic, you'll notice that it has a growl to it! In fact, when I listen to this area in a person's body, I can tell if they have a fierce critic, because the fork actually produces a growling sound. I can guarantee that if that voice were a person following you around, you wouldn't tolerate it! You'd punch them in the nose and tell them to scram. You wouldn't put up with someone else bullying you, and yet you are willing to tolerate it inside your own mind. You tolerate your inner critic because you believe on some level that A) you deserve it, and/or B) that you can abuse, punish, and berate yourself into health and beauty and success—no matter how many times this approach has failed in the past.

If you could hear how much dissonance the inner critic creates in your being, you would be appalled. What we really want is to be able to rest in this moment in contentment without feeling that there's anything wrong with us or the world around us. The inner critic robs us of that possibility. That state of contentment is the state in which everything in your body works! All your cells are functioning optimally. Your heart rate variability is groovy. Everything is humming along in your systems. When you get stressed, whether it comes from the outside or is self-inflicted, your whole system starts to go out of whack, and you actually energize viruses and pathogens in the system that thrive on chaos rather than order. This is one of the main reasons we get sick after periods of stress.

We want to honor our cells and allow them to do their thing, because when it comes right down to it, it is cellular health that determines overall health, and one way we can do that is by policing the voice of the inner critic that's creating noise in the signal and throwing the body into a state of stress. A simple way to do this is to create what I call a *note to self.* Imagine that you did something you shouldn't have done. It makes you feel terrible, and you beat yourself up. The guilt and shame follows you around and puts you through the wringer. Your mind just keeps circling back to the voice of, *Shouldn't have done that, shouldn't have done that, shouldn't have done that.*

That's when you create a note to self, which sounds something like this: *Okay, self, I'm making a mental note that next time I'm faced with a similar situation, I'll do my best to remember to do it this other way.* Maybe you'll take a moment to collect yourself before you press Send on that angry email. Maybe you'll think about your larger financial goals before you go on an online shopping spree. Whatever it is, just file it away as a note to yourself. Acknowledge what happened as a learning experience. Know that next time, you'll remember that pain and discomfort and seek to avoid it.

If the inner critic comes back and tries to give you shit again for your bad behavior, you can point to the note and say, "No, no, I got the point. I got the memo here. You don't need to keep telling me the same thing." The note is filed, this case is closed, goodbye. You don't allow the shame to keep coming and kicking and biting and scratching at you. It's much easier to move on when you've found the lesson and the actionable takeaway. Sink down into the discomfort, feel it, learn from it, forgive yourself, and then just move on.

Another strategy that's worked well for many of my students is to create the construct of an inner coach. When the inner critic starts "should-ing" all over you, you can say, *Thank you for the input, and I would like to know what my inner coach has to say.* The inner coach is kind and encouraging but also firm and resolute in making sure that you stick to your goals and do the work. The inner coach says, "Hey, did you get that note to self? Let's pay attention to that." Then there's none of that other bull-shit that weighs you down. You can let the inner critic run its program and say what it wants to say, but then turn instead to your inner coach and choose to listen to what they have to say. It's very hard to delete the program of the inner critic entirely, but over time and with practice, you hear from the critic less and less. It's helpful to have this other construct of a coach that we can give our energies to.

LEFT SIDE: FRUSTRATION AND DISAPPOINTMENT

The chaotic waveforms found on the left side of the sacral chakra relate to frustration and disappointment—in particular, frustration over unmet needs and unfulfilled desires.

Frustration and disappointment are often the result of feeling disconnected from our power in ways that we can't understand or seem to get to the root of. *Why am I creatively blocked? Why can't I find love? Why can't I make more money? Why can't I just be happy?* Often, it's interference that's been in our DNA for generations. We can't find the root and pull it up because it's so deeply buried in the system. I often find a tone here that feels "dead in the water." It's a sense of not really knowing what your passion and creativity is. When life force is denied and creative power is left unexpressed, frustration and disappointment are usually the result.

Again, we're dealing with the core issues of the left-hand ditch: Getting stuck in unmet needs and frustration around the things we're not doing, being, or having. Here it's specifically related to the money we want but don't have, the creativity we're not expressing, the intimacy and sexual fulfillment that's lacking, and the multitude of ways that we're just not enjoying our lives. That energy of frustration can go yang and rise up into the fiery anger of the solar plexus and liver/gallbladder, or it can go yin and sink down into a swampy sadness on the left side of the lower belly.

One of the most common constructs I encounter in this area is an old childhood pattern of retreating and internalizing. If we weren't receiving the love we need early on in life, especially at age seven and under, the natural response is to view ourselves as the cause. A child will conclude that the reason they're not getting love from Mom or Dad is because they're not good enough. That triggers a quiet disappointment and a diminishing of our energies over time. It's like a snail pulling into a shell; a retreating of the bright, overflowing energy of a child whose nature is to love everyone and everything. This happens to almost everyone in our culture to varying degrees, but it seems to happen more acutely to the more sensitive and empathic among us. There's a light, bright part of ourselves that steps into the shadows and goes off-line. When I see this in my clients, I invite them to extend compassion to their younger selves and send healing to whatever wounds were taken on as a result of those situations where they felt neglected, rejected, or denied love and connection. Send compassion and forgiveness to the people who participated in that retraction. It's easy to blame, but ultimately compassion, forgiveness, and understanding are what heal us.

Another pattern I have seen in this area in many people, myself included, is what I call the *posture of victimhood*. In this inner energetic arrangement, we are hunkered down in our left hips—frustrated over not being heard, not getting our needs met, and feeling like a powerless victim at the hands of some perpetrator or dictator in our lives.

Not that long ago, I found myself in this exact situation. It has been a familiar pattern to me as someone who was the youngest and smallest in most situations. As I have said, the tracks that get laid down early become the tracks of our lives. As I was fussing in my head about someone close to me who was giving me a hard time, I suddenly became aware of my energetic posture within my body, and sure enough, there I was, completely out of energetic balance. My knickers were clearly in a habitual twist as I was playing the same old tapes of powerlessness in my inner story. Armed with this self-awareness, I consciously used my mind to bring my inner energy flow back into the midline, stood up straight, and took a moment to settle into this more balanced inner experience. From this perspective of alignment, I reconsidered the situation and suddenly saw an approach to it that I hadn't previously considered, one that was win-win and took me out of the victim/perpetrator dynamic.

This is the trick: to not attach to these patterns and stories, and instead to step out of them into a new pattern, a new story. You don't need someone outside of yourself moving that energy with a tuning fork—you can do it yourself, from the inside out. Try it right now: Check in with your inner alignment. Explore how to use your mind to straighten yourself out from the inside out. Make it a regular practice, and you will be amazed at how just shifting your inner photonic composition changes your experience of yourself and your life.

BACK SIDE: RECEIVING PLEASURE AND ABUNDANCE

Every energy center has its theme of receiving that's connected to the back side of the chakra. I have found that most people are so programmed into giving and not receiving that the back sides of their chakras are closed up like little clams. The image I often see in the back of the sacral chakra is a dog with its tail between its legs. We want to untuck the tail and open up to receiving the abundance of gifts and pleasure that life is constantly offering. Do you allow yourself to receive simple pleasures? Do you feel worthy of enjoying good sex? Creative inspiration? Delicious food? Can you ask for a raise without feeling undeserving of it?

But I'm not just talking about sex or money. We can receive pleasure from the scent of a rose, a beautiful birdsong, the warmth of the sun on our faces, a smile from a stranger. These simple sensory pleasures, these little blessings of life, are available to us all the time if only we believe that we are worthy of receiving them.

If we want abundance in our lives, we have to be willing to claim that, to start tapping into the abundance that's already all around us. In nature, you put one seed in the ground, and it can bear thousands of fruits. All the stars in the sky and all the cells in your body, there's no lack or shortage! You being in that abundant flow doesn't take anything away from anyone else—in fact, the opposite is true. The more we receive good things, the more we become channels for them. It's a beautiful thing to have the resources to help ourselves and others. It's wonderful to be able to take care of our children, partners, and parents, to treat our friends, and to contribute to the causes we care about. It feels fantastic to be able to buy art and support artists!

Think about what you receive in every moment as a precious gift from life itself: the breath! At every moment, nature is supplying you with vital energy that keeps you alive and fuels you in everything you want and need to do. The tendency to hold the breath is deeply connected to the tendency to block ourselves from receiving. If you're not allowing yourself to receive the life force that comes in through the breath, then how are you going to receive pleasure, love, and money?

Try consciously breathing in light. Imagine a golden fluid light flooding from your lungs to your whole being. Let yourself be inwardly bathed in the same electricity that powers the sun and the stars. On the inhale, let the breath flow joyously to every cell in your body. Let yourself be with the delight of receiving nature's goodness and allowing it to energize you. Be kind to your cells. You'd never say that your cells aren't worthy of the resources they need to function properly!

COMING HOME TO YOUR PLEASURE BODY

Here's an interesting idea to consider while working with your sacral chakra: Your human body was exquisitely designed by life itself to experience and enjoy pleasure. You have a *pleasure body,* and it's the opposite of your pain body. Life evolves by moving away from pain and toward pleasure. Pleasure is a big part of what life is all about! Anything and everything we do or want, from eating chocolate to seeking enlightenment, is because it's going to bring us pleasure. We are set up to get a tremendous amount of pleasure from our eyes, ears, mouths, and noses, from our skin and reproductive areas. Nature gave us these senses to take in and appreciate the delights of creation, from orgasms to beautiful sunsets. We're not meant to live life from our pain bodies. We were made to experience the wonders of creation through our biological pleasure bodies.

This notion of pleasure as the whole purpose of our biological beings might sound "unspiritual" to some folks. When I was talking about all of this with my friend Marci, she said, "But, Eileen, what about enlightenment? What about the bliss of the union with the divine? Isn't that what we're built for?" To which I responded, "Well, that sounds pretty darn pleasurable to me."

Everything we want, everything we desire and are motivated toward, is going to give us pleasure in some way or another. It's just faulty programming and incoherent waveforms that convince us that there's something bad or wrong about that pursuit of pleasure. Our Puritan upbringing and all these stories we have around spirituality and self-improvement tell us, "No, no, no, I've got to be good. I have to eat clean and sit in silence and control my desires." Meanwhile, we're missing out on so much of the beauty and joy of this earthly human experience.

Often connected to our stories about health, spirituality, and "doing good" in the world, there is a mind virus that tells us that pleasure is selfish and bad somehow and, therefore, that we should feel guilty for enjoying it. In the quest to become a more enlightened being, many of us deny ourselves the pleasures of this human experience that is happening right now. Pleasure is messy, it's animalistic, it's "lower chakra." We just want to focus on love and light and ascend to the heavens! We want to concentrate on the upper chakras, to be "good," to deny ourselves chocolate and wine and coffee. We want to serve and be compassionate. There is so much suffering in the world, so therefore, we should be suffering, too. How dare we enjoy sex or a decadent meal while the sixth mass extinction is going on around us! I've been seeing this more and more, and my response is that stories in the media aren't a good reason to not appreciate the taste of a fresh strawberry. We can still enjoy pleasure while the world is falling apart, and indeed, we *should*. Taking part in healthy pleasures raises our own light and coherence, which brings more light and coherence into the collective electromagnetic body.

I know that the more I nourish myself through receiving pleasure and beauty, the more my own needs are met, and the more I can serve and uplift others. Repeat after me: *Pleasure is not selfish.* When you avail yourself of beauty and pleasure, you're much happier and more content. You radiate a more coherent vibe and have a positive impact on the people around you. The more time you spend in your pleasure body, the better for you and the rest of us. Making sure that your organism is content and not in a state of need is important! When you're in a state of lack and need, you're like a free radical. You're just taking and absorbing from everything around you, and it makes you hard to be around. But when you're satisfied, you become like a walking Himalayan salt lamp, radiating good vibes all around you.

THE PLEASURABLE PATH TO GOOD HEALTH

At one of my recent workshops, a student raised her hand and asked me, "What kind of spiritual teacher are you? You swear, drink beer and coffee, and eat meat and chocolate." My response was that spirituality and pleasure are not mutually exclusive, and I also don't consider myself a spiritual teacher—I am interested in the full spectrum of being human, not just the "spiritual" aspects. I am a firm believer that we can enjoy pleasure while we're getting healthy and enlightened.

Guilt, shame, and self-denial are not a sustainable path to good health. I advocate what I call *moderate hedonism* as an approach to enjoying pleasures without sacrificing your health and energy levels. Health is my number-one pursuit, but no food is off limits to me. I let myself enjoy anything and everything in the right dose without guilt.

It can take a little time and some self-awareness to get there. My husband is going through this process now. He used to be what I'd call an extreme hedonist: he loves pleasure, and for much of his life, he overdid it on things like coffee, ice cream, and beer. When he hit forty, all of a sudden, his body wouldn't put up with it anymore. He had to go in the opposite direction and give up everything—which was not easy for him! Today, he's in a recovery place where he is starting to be able to reintroduce some pleasurable things. My goal is to help him aim for successful moderate hedonism where he can enjoy the things that give him pleasure without craving or overindulging in them.

If you're dealing with some health challenge or pattern of addiction and need to restrict what you consume for a period of time, I encourage you to do that. In my own pursuit of health, I had to go through giving up all sugar and sweeteners for months to clear out a stubborn candida overgrowth and to overcome my own cravings for it. I've quit pretty much everything at some point or another, just to make sure I was not using any of it compulsively anymore. It took me a long time to master moderate hedonism (decades, actually), but now that I have, there is great freedom in being able to enjoy everything in the appropriate amounts.

I'd like to suggest that you, too, are capable of enjoying the pleasure of good food and self-nourishment. We can get healthy with the aim of coming to a place of balance. We really need to hold the vision that moderation is possible. This is supreme idealism, and the premise might not work for everyone, depending on your patterns of addiction and how deeply they run—but I'm not going to come from any other place, because that is what has worked for me, as well as the people around me who also follow this approach to life.

Moderate hedonism at its core says that we are truly able to enjoy pleasures in a healthy way when we've freed ourselves from our compulsions about them. That's the work here. It's really the path of the tortoise: slow and steady rather than all or nothing. Any time we go after anything with any kind of compulsion, what we're doing is treating the emotions underneath the craving. The change starts with self-awareness. Check in with yourself: *Am I wanting this chocolate cake because I am going after it compulsively to soothe some uncomfortable feeling?* If the answer is no, then ask yourself, *Can my system tolerate this piece of chocolate cake? How much of this pleasurable substance can I successfully metabolize in this moment?* Maybe two bites is all. Another day, maybe it's fine to eat the full slice, because you can feel that your digestive fire is burning bright enough.

I enjoy in the range of three to five alcoholic drinks a week but very rarely have more than one per night. When my two international class coordinators, Kimberly Schipke and Jessica Luibrand, and I were teaching a course in England recently, we had a powerful session one afternoon. That evening after class, it was a two-cocktail night for all of us, and the two of them rarely drink. We went out to a nice restaurant and had two cocktails because that was just the right thing to do in that moment. If we hadn't been in the right frame of mind, those drinks might not have sat well. But we were in a frame of mind where two cocktails just hit the spot, and we didn't experience any ill effects.

You have to learn to pay attention to these subtle cues. It's about getting back to wild eating. Wild animals don't overeat! They eat when they're hungry and stop when they're full. Period! We as humans need to trust our own inner senses to tell us what we need to do, and that is a process. If you keep at it, you recognize the subtle cue that when your tongue stops enjoying what you're eating, that's a sign that you're full. It's about learning to recognize those very subtle things. When we're in this overly yang, overthinking and overdoing, sugar-craving mode, we're not exquisitely attuned to the subtle cues of our bodies. But the more you learn to breathe and ground, to hang out in your central axis, to pay attention to the moment, the more you can hear the cues.

What it really comes down to is mastering the pain-pleasure threshold. For me, one cappuccino in the morning is pleasure, but two is pain (not only for me but for everyone around me because I'm all cranked up!). As much as I love my cappuccino, I love one more than I love two. We all have to figure out through trial and error how to stay in the pleasure zone and to love and respect ourselves enough to stay on the inside of that boundary. But if you do overstep it, don't go into inner critic mode. Give yourself a note to self to check in next time. Don't make some all-or-nothing rule. Just make the commitment to check in with yourself next time to find what's really appropriate for you in the moment.

12

SOLAR PLEXUS:
Your Radiant Inner Sun

In November of 2019, I conducted a group Biofield Tuning session at the Sacred Science of Sound, founded by Jeralyn Glass, conference in Los Angeles. When I do this sort of thing, I stand up in front of the crowd and envision a hologram of the group. I wave my tuning forks through the air, and in doing so, I can actually read and adjust the energy of the group. (Yes, I know this sounds far-out, but I honestly wouldn't do such weird things if they didn't produce outcomes!) I call out each zone, and the group energy of that particular zone gets reflected in the tone of the fork. I stay with it until it shifts, and then I move on. In this particular session, we were going through the entire body, starting at the feet, and we were moving along nicely until I got to the right side of the solar plexus. This is the zone in the biofield anatomy that holds information related to the emotion of anger, as well as our relationships with our fathers.

Despite repeated strikes with an assortment of different forks, the energy refused to budge and come to a clear tone.

"C'mon, people," I said, glancing at the clock. "This is your inner light! We need to let it shine!"

The energy still wasn't moving, so I asked folks to share things that were blocking their lights from shining. Response after response popcorned out into the room. I couldn't believe how many reasons there were. Fear of judgment, fear of persecution, fear of not being good enough—the list went on and on! While the energy started to loosen a bit, talking about it wasn't enough to get things to clear. The whole group had to stand up, make sound, shake their bodies around. Spontaneously, the group broke out into singing "This Little Light of Mine" together. Once all that happened, the tone finally came in loud and clear, and we were able to proceed and finish up all the other centers.

This experience really speaks to me of the greater cultural picture of the solar plexus. We have been conditioned to feel powerless and disconnected, to suppress our anger, to hide our light. Deeply ingrained patterns throughout millennia and maybe even lifetimes have dimmed us out, and we are afraid, many for very good reasons, to shine! Not being fully present and engaged in this center can deprive us of the full extent of our power and potential.

The solar plexus, located just above the navel, is our radiant inner sun. It resonates with the frequency of the color yellow, the vowel sound "oh," and the seed syllable "RAM." It is a vital and information-filled energy center, with a whole council of intelligent organs working together. On the right side, you've got the liver, gallbladder, right kidney, and right adrenal, and on the left, you have the spleen, pancreas, stomach, left kidney, and left adrenal. In the years I spent exploring and mapping the body and the biofield anatomy, I came to have a great appreciation for the solar plexus—and a singular respect for the liver. In Chinese medicine, the liver is seen as the general of the army that is the body. It oversees all operations. People debate about whether the heart or the brain is the seat of consciousness, but I've come to see it as the liver, as the ancient Greeks did. Your liver is paying attention to everything! It attends to your respiration, circulation, digestion, and elimination with exquisite attention and care.

Emotionally, we store anger and powerlessness in this center, as well as self-esteem, personal power, and the energies of our mothers and fathers. This area contains so much information that it seems to me that there may be another kind of electromagnetic axis here. It took me many years to be able to differentiate the different tones and frequencies I was finding in this region.

The gut is often called the *second brain,* but from what I've seen, it could almost be the primary brain (I mean, the small intestine *looks* like the brain!). When we strengthen this energy center and learn to operate from our cores, we unlock a huge amount of discipline, focus, determination, clarity, and personal power. We're able to set goals and achieve them. We can move forward with projects all the way to the end. We're able to assert ourselves in a way that's healthy and effective. We interface with other people's energies in a way that's diplomatic, and we set strong boundaries. We also enjoy a strong digestive fire. So much of what I see in people who struggle with food allergies, gas, bloating, and acid reflux is an excess of personal power that's locked up and stuck out on the sides of the solar plexus. The digestive fire, which should be strong and hearty, gets weakened and diffused.

When the energy of the solar plexus is gathered, it's miraculous. It's phenomenal what we can do with it. But when the energy here is scattered, our wills and personal power are weakened. The left side holds the yin imbalance of *powerlessness.* Here, I find a person's relationship with their mother—connected to the spleen and pancreas—as well as the nurturance they received in childhood and their ability to properly nourish and care for themselves. The right-side, yang imbalance is related to *anger* (toward ourselves and others) and our relationships with our fathers. In line with many holistic traditions, including Chinese medicine and Ayurveda, I've found anger to be processed and stored in the liver.

Who we are is unimaginably powerful. That's our nature. But our wills and personal power become weakened because so much of our solar plexus energy gets stuck on either side of the center: in anger, powerlessness, unresolved issues with our mothers and fathers, unhealthy eating habits, and adrenal glands that are running like a toilet with a broken handle. The energy gets siphoned off by difficult characters around us because we don't have strong boundaries. Fundamentally, anger and powerlessness are both unsuccessful expressions of power. But when we get into the center of the solar plexus, there's a smooth functionality to how we exert our energies and take action in the world.

Around ten inches off the solar plexus in either direction are two energetic structures about the size of a hockey puck that I call the *mother* and *father zones.* We are all strongly informed by the energy of our parents. It lives on either side of our solar plexus and is always affecting our fields. Even if the parents are long dead, the history of that relationship is alive. I can stick a fork in the father zone and tell you all about the personality of your dad. It's all encoded there. Often, I come into contact with structures here that feel like energetic walls, which happens when people shut out their parents. Those structures can really decrease the functioning of the liver and gallbladder on the right/dad side and spleen and pancreas on the left/mother side by blocking the flow of energy, and it can even move into the kidney, adrenals, and stomach. Creating strong boundaries, but not walls, is a key part of the work of cultivating a healthy solar plexus.

The back of the solar plexus relates to receiving support. Did you receive support from your parents? Are you supporting yourself? Are you paying your bills and getting enough sleep? Being open here is about getting the resources we need from other people, ourselves, the universe, and the flow of nature. We're getting all the things we need to move forward with the flow of our intentions. That can be very simple. When a stranger holds a door open for you, you can receive and have gratitude for that support. When the universe provides the perfect parking spot for you, you're being supported. You can change the script, open the portal, and let that support come in. We get all shut down here when we're walking around with a story that we never get the support we need. Then you're not even going to notice when support is trying to come in, because you're too wrapped up in your story. We want to open that up and really let this support into our bodies. The mantra here is: *I am open to receiving support. The more support I receive, the more support I can give. I am supported.*

YOUR RADIANT INNER SUN

When people start exploring the world of energy, they tend to get stars in their eyes around the heart chakra. A lot of New Age practices have this idea of operating from your heart center, which can be useful but also limiting. Here's why I say that: When we get into the heart, there are so many layers of other things going on. There's hate. There's despair. There's depression. There's sadness. There's resentment. There's grief. We want to get to the love that's there, but it's like there are all these overlays on top of it. I find that anchoring your awareness in your heart can also have a rather top-heavy quality to it. It's not fully in your center.

The more that I work with energy, the more I become identified with my solar plexus. As a place to rest our awareness, I personally find the solar plexus to be much more peaceful and radiant than the heart. My experience is that when I'm anchored in my core, there's this easy suspension, just like the sun is suspended in the sky, and it spins around and spreads its light. The more you associate with your own inner sun, the more you end up in the flow of your natural orbit. Your digestive fire is stronger. Your mind is clear, and your intention is strong. That power, then, supports and lifts the heart. Trying to live from the heart when you're not supported from below just isn't as energy efficient. I think we want to occupy this golden ball of light in the very center of our beings and to allow that to flow up the central channel and energize the heart.

A common misperception about the solar plexus is that it is an overly yang, assertive, and ambitious energy. It's actually flowing rather than efforting or striving or pushing outward. When you're anchored in your central sun, the whole power of the universe is moving through you. A healthy will is a beautiful balance of yin and yang. It's an effortless surrender to the will of the universe. You're doing the work and taking steps to accomplish tasks, but there's not a sense of struggle about it. You do without doing, and everything gets done.

Take a moment to tune in to the frequency of the golden luminescence within you. As you drop further into the center of your being, feel your own inner radiance expanding out in every direction. Call back your power and vitality. Use your intention to feed your inner furnace, stoking it up good and hot. Tell yourself that you're going to channel that power into effective action. Where does this new energy here want to go? How does it want to express itself?

RIGHT SIDE: FATHER, ANGER, LIVER AND GALLBLADDER, RIGHT KIDNEY, AND ADRENAL

The right side of the solar plexus holds information related to your father and your relationship with him, ancestral information from your paternal lineage, as well as the emotions of anger and blame. The energy here can be very hot, and I've often broken out in a sweat while working in this part of the field.

Ideally, the energy of the father is empowering and stabilizing. It's a reflection of our own solar element that mirrors our own brilliance back to us. If your father suffered trauma or for whatever reason wasn't in touch with those aspects of himself, that empowering influence will be lacking. If his energy was unstable, then there's a destabilizing element here. It often feels to me like pieces that are meant to stack neatly on top of one another that got misaligned, creating a fundamental structural weakness. That influence creates a structural weakness both in the physiology, especially in the spine and mid-back, and also in the vibrational weave of the solar plexus. This is common in people who had fathers who were alcoholics or rageoholics or for other reasons were not functional in their own beings or in their relationships with their children.

I've been consistently surprised by just how many issues I find when working in the father zone. A lot of us had fathers who were defensive or unyielding or rigid. Others grew up with fathers who weren't physically present or emotionally available. That creates a sort of gap. *I'm not connecting with Dad. He's just not there. Where is he? He's at work. He's gone behind a newspaper or TV show.* Another common pattern is fathers who were angry, volatile, or unpredictable, which has a huge impact on the highly sensitive developing nervous system. Lack of support from the father seems to particularly impact the gallbladder. Virtually everyone I have ever worked on with gallbladder issues, including having had it removed, all had extremely challenging relationships with their fathers.

Anger gets stored in the liver. It's a very fiery, hot emotion that creates a lot of problems when it's internalized. We go numb with the power of this emotion because we don't know how to express it. When we suppress anger, we suppress fire, which has very much to do with our vitality. When we don't fully express and release our anger (and many of us don't), it gets stuck and causes problems in our livers and digestive systems.

When we don't express our anger, over time, we end up stupefying the liver. That's where those molecules of anger go and hang out. The barrage of suppressed anger, stress, toxins, alcohol and drug use, and other environmental influences create a very difficult time for our livers and consequently our consciousness. People with anger that they don't know what to do with often reach for what I call *liver pacifiers*: sugar, excessive carbs, alcohol, chocolate, and dense dairy products like ice cream or cheese. These things are fine in moderation, but in excess, they clog the liver. As I've mentioned, I used to have a terrible, uncontrollable sugar addiction. And all the while I was eating so much sugar, I was telling myself, *I never get angry.* I didn't even realize at the time that I was using sugar to dampen my anger. I couldn't understand why I couldn't seem to quit sugar, but it was because I was using it to cover up all the anger that I wasn't ready to face. I've also found that people who have difficult relationships with their fathers (which is surprisingly many of us) tend to repress the tough feelings associated with this using liver pacifiers.

We need to figure out how it feels best for us to release our anger, whether it's through physical exertion or scrubbing the bathtub or drumming or writing or speaking our truth diplomatically. Anger shows up for me as a staccato frequency, and it seems to want to move in jerky ways. Getting down on your knees and scrubbing the floor or the bathtub is a great thing to do to get that waveform to move through you. I also like the affirmation: *I give myself permission to figure out how to express my anger appropriately.* Once we start letting go of our backlogs of anger, once we start noticing where we're holding grievances and seek to rectify them, our relationship with anger changes. We soften out of it. We're less likely to react to a situation with anger, or if we do, it spurs us to meaningful action and we resolve the problem. Anger stops accumulating and flaring when we've addressed that backlog and allowed the anger to exist as a part of us.

Here's the thing about anger: It's a propellant. We don't want to wash away our anger. It serves the honorable purpose of moving us into constructive action. Anger about the state of politics might move you to run for local office. Or you're angry about mass incarceration, so you donate to organizations that are fighting for change there. If you're angry at someone who is treating you with disrespect, you might be moved to speak your truth. I was angry that a food addiction hijacked my life, and that drove me to figure out how to solve the problem and in turn help others. I'm moved to use the tools and knowledge that I have acquired to help people feel better. Let your anger propel you to some kind of action that pushes the dial in a positive direction.

What we don't want is to just get stuck in anger and powerlessness with no effective action. If you're getting angry at the state of the world and not doing anything about it, then you're just wasting gas. I see this happen all the time with politics and environmental issues. I'm not saying that we shouldn't get angry about what's going on out there—we should. But we want to let those energies move us to effective action performed with compassion, kindness, respect, and love. It's about coming back to the central channel and moving from a posture of presence. When you're getting stuck on the sides of the solar plexus, then you're spinning back and forth between anger and powerlessness. We want to instead use that anger to propel us back to center and move into action from there.

LEFT SIDE: MOTHER, POWERLESSNESS, SPLEEN AND PANCREAS, LEFT KIDNEY, AND ADRENAL

When I was first figuring out the biofield anatomy, I had to take some real time to reflect on what word I would give to the vibrational imbalance on the left side of the solar plexus. What it sounded like to me, as strange as it sounds, was *the present tense of regret*. What would you call regret as it's occurring in the moment? I came to realize that it was powerlessness. *I was powerless to walk away from that toxic relationship. I was powerless to digest that big meal. I was powerless over my addiction. I was powerless to act on my dreams*. It's the feeling that's created when we feel that we don't have the inner or outer resources in the moment to execute our desired outcomes.

One phenomenon I often encounter here is energy that's moving backward rather than forward. People whose wills have been overrun by other people, or whose parents suppressed their spirits, will often go into life with a pattern of being a doormat and having other people impressing their wills upon them habitually. There's a weak will that was broken or damaged in childhood. This often has an inherited element, especially for women, who have historically been forced to play second fiddle and have their wills overridden by men. That creates feelings of powerlessness and weakness, as well as an inability to digest and manage experiences and to metabolize other people's energy. It can also give rise to the experience of heartburn or acid reflux, as other people impress their wills on us.

Part of the story of powerlessness, often rooted in the mother, is a pattern of worry, fretting, and inaction. Instead of taking constructive action, we go around in this circular swirling energy of worry instead. We get stuck in the left-hand ditch in our stories of victimhood. This script can be flipped by recognizing powerlessness as a habit. It's just a pattern. The story might have been going on for generations in your female lineage, but it can be reprogrammed. Even as you're reading this, you can consciously use your mind to pull your energy back. All the places you've given away power, all the places you saw your mom give away power. Pull it back, rein it in, own it, claim it, radiate it. Cry if you need to and then pull it back in some more.

Here we also find the mother zone and the record of your mother's energy and your relationship with her dating back to conception. I've observed in many people a consistent pattern of maternal stress and over-whelm. So many of our mothers were unduly stressed, raising children with too much responsibility and too much isolation. Historically, it took a village to raise a child. Earlier generations had extended family around with grandparents, aunts, and uncles there to help. It's really not natural for a woman to raise children without familial and community support, and yet many of our mothers lacked any semblance of the support system they needed. When a mother is isolated, it takes a toll on her mental and emotional health. For the child, that energy creates a layer of noise on the outer boundary of the field that impacts their whole being.

Another very damaging pattern in the mother zone is the frequency of postpartum depression. If your mother went into a depressive state after going through pregnancy, labor, and delivery, that tone of sadness, isolation, and exhaustion will show up as a pattern in your own field. A baby is a little resonance machine, and they will pick up on and recipro- cate the vibrations around them, especially from their mothers. I always advise my students and clients to learn their birth stories. What was go- ing on with your mom while you were in the womb? What was your birth like? What was happening at home when you were an infant? Ask your mother, if she's still alive, or check in with another family member if she's not around anymore. When you know the story, you can work through it. You can start to change the impact you've carried with you from that experience—and we *all* carry things around from the begin- ning of our lives.

My own mother was thirty-nine years old when she got pregnant with me. Early on in the pregnancy, her doctors told her that I had Down syndrome and that I'd only have one leg. She already had her hands more than full with five kids and went through her pregnancy worrying about how she was going to manage having a special-needs child in the mix. Thankfully, I was born healthy, but carried with me a strange sense that I was deficient in some way and that there was something wrong with me for a very long time. It took a fair amount of work to back those imprints out of my system—but it is absolutely possible to do.

The energy of the mother directly influences the spleen, which plays a very maternal role in our systems: the work of drawing nourishment from the food we eat and using it to build healthy blood and immunity. Both the spleen and the pancreas relate to our ability to nourish ourselves and to absorb the sweetness from life, with the pancreas regulating our blood sugar. If Mom wasn't sweet and nourishing, we end up with un- met needs and frustrated desires. If for whatever reason we didn't get the nurturing we needed from our mothers, we'll create stories of lack around that. When those needs aren't being met, we tell ourselves, "I'm not expecting that anymore. I don't care because I didn't get it and I never will." The result is a hardening up of the functioning of those organs. We stop being open to the sweetness of life. We stop nourishing ourselves emotionally and physically.

All of this is not to place further undue blame on our mothers (our culture does enough of that!). Mothering is an extremely difficult job under the best of circumstances. Part of our work here is forgiving our mothers for whatever we wanted or needed in childhood that we weren't able to receive from them, for whatever reason. Almost everyone, even those with loving, healthy, and engaged mothers, has a story of lack somewhere around the mother zone. Even if your mother was hard to love, you don't really know her story. You don't know her inputs, and you don't know her story of redemption. *One of the biggest things I have learned from this work is that the only sentiment that is logical, reasonable, and appropriate to extend to anyone is* compassion, *first and foremost to yourself and then radiating out from there.* That's a manifestation of a healthy solar plexus.

Dropping out of judgment and into compassion is a relief. It's not easy, but, man, does it lighten our loads. There are some old emotions and stories that you'll have to work through to get there, but once you get there, it becomes a lot easier and more natural. Let's choose to radiate compassionate blessings to others rather than to cast judgment or feel like a victim of someone else's incoherence.

BOUNDARIES: GOOD FENCES MAKE GOOD NEIGHBORS

The most common manifestations of the left-side imbalance of powerlessness are weak boundaries and a pattern of being taken advantage of. There's often a rip or tear in the double-layer membrane of the biofield in this area where energy leaks out. It's a vague and leaky and weak area—which can manifest physically as leaky gut syndrome. It's an experience of being permeable where you don't want to be permeable. You're giving too much of yourself away, pouring your energy out, and not having clear boundaries to protect yourself.

Boundary violations by parents or other authority figures early in life create patterns where we end up violating our own boundaries, through poor health habits or any other lack of self-care or self-respect—thus reinforcing a familiar pattern of powerlessness and a disconnection from our own wills.

When I work with my students and clients on healing boundary issues, I tend to focus on strengthening the central channel rather than the actual outer boundary. This seems to be an easier and more accessible way of getting the job done. The central channel *is* the outer boundary of the field. The energy of that central axis flows out through the head and feet and circles around the outer perimeter of the biofield. That means that the more you're aligned with your axis—the more centered you are in your electromagnetic core—the stronger that outer boundary becomes. The outer membrane of your biofield is just like a cell membrane; when a cell has high voltage, it's in a state of optimal functioning. It lets in what it wants to let in, and it lets out what it wants to let out. The cell has sufficient energy to manage that inflow and outflow of information. But when the voltage drops, things get in that shouldn't be getting in. And then things leak out that shouldn't get out. We become susceptible to pathogens and viruses and bacteria and energy vampires because we don't have the defenses to keep up a strong boundary. The more we strengthen our electromagnetic core, the more we raise our voltage, the stronger that outer boundary becomes. We have the *energy* necessary to recognize and assert our boundaries.

As we become more centered, stronger boundaries are the natural result. Healthy boundaries are a win-win; they keep our relationships thriving and mutually beneficial. Good fences make good neighbors! We don't want to feel like our houses are full of guests who have overstayed their welcome. We don't want to feel like people are sucking and feeding on our energies, and then that we are also somehow doing this to ourselves within our own bodies. When you live like this, you become vulnerable to things like autoimmune diseases because your immune system is weakened. Your defenses are down! Your voltage drops, and you become vulnerable to pathogens—or the body gets confused about who's the invader, and it starts attacking itself. When I was in a place in my life where I was giving everything away to everyone else, as well as three months pregnant, I got ehrlichiosis, a fierce tick-borne disease— sort of like Lyme on steroids—that almost killed me. It knocked me flat for months, during which time I was forced to finally give myself the care and attention I had been giving away to everyone else in my life.

Boundary issues are often connected to the heart chakra, which carries the imbalance of over-caretaking and putting others' needs before our own, as well as the throat, which has to do with our ability to speak our own needs and desires. Being able to say no is huge. If you don't honor the needs of your organism, your organism will break down. You need to be able to recognize your own needs and to know when you're putting them aside to seek approval or be accommodating or get love. This is real self-care—not just eating kale and meditating but creating strong personal boundaries and advocating for our own needs.

RECLAIMING OUR POWER

To have a strong and balanced solar plexus, we need to come into a clean and clear perception of our own power. That requires a process of rooting through the old beliefs and stories we have around power. Many of us have negative associations with the word *power*. Often, we believe that it's bad. We believe, erroneously, that any power is inherently power *over* others. One of the big things I see all the time that causes people to shut down their own personal power is the fear of misusing that power. I can't tell you how many spiritual folks have said to me, "I was really powerful in a past life, but I abused my power, and now I'm skittish around owning my power." This is a story that I do not indulge. I tell them that this is a story that may or may not be true, but in either case, it is not serving them.

Let's just bust the myth right now that you're going to misuse your power. If you are reading this book, it is likely that you are here for good. There's no reason to be afraid that you're going to take power and use it over other people. That's not how we're going to associate with power. We're going to use our power to support and uplift others, to make a difference in the planet for good, to add coherence and functionality and sanity to the mix. If the world is full of people who want to do good but think power is bad, then nothing is going to happen. If you came here to be on Team Earth because you want to help improve the situation on the planet, then you being powerless is not helping.

Let's make it less scary. A simple definition of power is *energy*. It's your horsepower. It's *strength*. More power means more ability to get the job done, whatever that job is. If you were stronger than you are right now—if you went from a 60-watt bulb to a 100-watt bulb—suddenly, you'd have more energy to get things done in your life, to finish projects, to manage difficult characters, to bust that clutter, to kick pathogens out of your cells. Power is voltage and light and lumens. Why wouldn't you want that? It's your job to get stronger and brighter for the benefit of all, most of all yourself! Whether you have more power to get through the day with more grace and humor as a caregiver, or to steer a large business successfully, or jump higher, or run faster, we all benefit from having more available energy.

There's no way you can misuse your light. When it's true power, you're not going to use it to dominate other people. If you're dominating others, then you're operating from fear, not power. True power is the power to support and uplift yourself and everyone else. It's the power to shine light in other people's lives and in the dark corners of your own psyche and your ancestral inheritances. Power is the ability to lighten your own load so that you're better able to fulfill your purpose or, at the very least, just be healthier. It's about turning up your own wattage and being brighter! What on earth is dangerous or scary or bad about that?

Power allows us to live our gifts. We know what our gifts are, and we take action to develop those gifts and get them out into the world. We've all experienced how moving it is to see someone who's free and empowered to live their gifts. I once saw a viral video of this high school senior in Massachusetts who was an incredible artist and drew charcoal portraits of each of the 419 students in his graduating class. On the last week of school, he came in early and hung them up in the walls of the hallway. People cried when they saw these beautiful portraits. This is a perfect example of someone who is fully engaged in their solar plexus and has a healthy relationship to their own power. He had a vision, and he did the work to act it out. He had a gift that he developed and shared in a way that made a difference in other people's lives.

OVERCOMING 80 PERCENT SYNDROME

On a more fundamental level, power just helps us to *get things done*. We set goals and achieve them. We complete tasks and finish projects. We execute on our dreams and visions. Wherever you're missing the mark in your life, there is a lack of power. If you had more power—and if you had a strong belief and inner experience of increased power—you wouldn't be stuck spinning your wheels. Think about all the places where you're not hitting the target in your life. Maybe you're not getting it together financially and you feel powerless around money. Or maybe you don't know your purpose or mission in life, and you feel powerless there. Whatever it is, more power—more voltage in your system and strength in your core—is the thing that will get you to where you want to be.

Eighty percent syndrome is our propensity to start a project and get pretty far with it, but fail to see it through to the very end. I see this all the time in people with a weak solar plexus, often those who have a lot of stuck energy related to one or both parents. Their lives are littered with unfinished projects (and often, frustrated partners). The reason we fall short is because we've got too much energy stuck in the alcoholic dad and the powerless mom, in ancestral stories, bad food, and disempowering self-talk. There are so many reasons why we don't have enough focus and energy in the solar plexus—all these factors are spreading the energy out all over the place and we can't access it.

When we free up the energy of our solar center, we find the chutzpah and gumption to go that extra mile to the finish line. And it feels *amazing*. If you're only going 80 percent, you're making investments and you're not getting a return on them. I was a big 80 percenter for much of my life, but I finally realized that when I wrap something up, I feel great, and when I leave something partway done, I feel crummy because that thing is still in my system consuming my energy. I promise you: *The return on investment of going the last mile is way worth it.* It's a mental block when we get to the last 10 or 20 percent and we tell ourselves that we can't do it. Those extra steps are not nearly as hard as we think they are. It's really just about creating a new habit of finishing what we've started. We can start small! Put the laundry in the drawer instead of leaving it in a stack on top of the dresser. Clean the last two pans left in the sink. Wherever we're leaving things off, just take the extra couple of steps. Finishing what we set out to do, even with the simplest things, creates a perception of our own power that generates an embodied experience of more power. Fortune favors the bold, and we will magnetize the things we want from moving into bold action.

And know that you'll feel amazing when it's done! Your solar plexus will be bright and glowing with satisfaction. I love the feeling of accomplishment. It's wonderful to tie a bow on something and call it done. It's a high! It activates the brain's reward system, and we're wired to reap the benefits. Don't deny yourself that good feeling.

When you're really feeling stuck, there's a visualization I use for honing will and intention. First, center your awareness in your inner sun. Then imagine a light beam that extends all the way out the front of that orb to penetrate the outer front edge of the field. This is an open channel for your intention to flow out and for information that's vital for you to receive to flow in. With this laser beam of focused intention, you're able to act with ease. You're able to move forward with a clear vision and powerful will. Imagine this golden yellow laserlike beam emerging from just above your navel and extending to the outer edge of your field. It's focused. It's getting all the way to the edge—not dropping off somewhere in the middle or getting pushed backward. It's getting to completion. It's getting all the way to where you need it to go. Feel into that sense of focus and confidence.

One thing to note: It took until I was fifty for me to realize that if I was kicking a particular can down the road and just not getting to it, it was something I needed help with. I learned that if I enlisted someone to help me with it, getting it done got a lot easier. When I was explaining this to my eighteen-year-old son, he told me that he didn't feel worthy of receiving help. This is a common sentiment, so check in to see if you also have that mind virus running. Gracious receiving gives dignity to the act of giving. It's okay to need help.

STOKING THE DIGESTIVE FIRE

Physically, a strong solar plexus means a strong digestive fire. When the energy that's gotten stuck on the sides of the field comes back to center, our inner fires are fed and fueled.

Robust digestion and elimination is one of the most important factors in our overall health. We want our digestive processes to be smooth sailing. That's a big part of why the solar plexus and the sacral center, which relate to our lower and upper digestive tracts, are so critical to the integrity and function of our system as a whole.

People with a lot of personal power are hearty digesters! They can digest and assimilate all kinds of things. If your digestive fire is hot enough, you can combust things like gluten and dairy without a problem.

I think of my digestive tract as an electrical incinerator. It turns calories into heat and inner light. The more powerful your inner incinerator, the better your digestion. My fire is so hot that it happily incinerates things like cheese, meat, and grains without a problem. If I'm going to eat a croissant, I just incinerate it. I burn it up in my inner furnace and turn it back into light—without any stories or guilt or judgment about it. I like to imagine that my fire is so hot that it can burn up any herbicides or pesticides or other pollutants that the food might be carrying. I know I can count on the little electrogenic organisms in my gut to help break down and burn up everything I consume.

Since I have to eat on the road a lot, this philosophy has been a game changer. Given the choice, I'll always take local, organic, small-farm foods. However, I don't always have that choice. No matter what I'm eating, I bless the food, the water in the food, and every person who handled it to get it to my plate, as well as their families. I enjoy it with gusto, and I burn it up with my healthy, energized digestive fire. Zero guilt and zero judgment about it being "good" or "bad" or "clean." I'm able to eat pizza, ice cream, doughnuts, french fries, cheese—or whatever fast food might be available in a midwestern airport. But I eat these things in relatively small amounts and only when I sense that my fire is up for the job.

While it's true that you are what you eat, it's also important to remember that a calorie is technically just a unit of heat. The digestive system distributes heat and light to our bodies. Another way to think of it is that your stomach is a woodstove and the food you eat is the wood. As long as you have a good base of coals—a strong and coherent inner fire plus hunger—you can toss in most anything, and it will burn well. It will help the fire burn stronger and brighter, distributing greater light and energy across the system. That said, an endless supply of junk will gum up most systems over time.

When the solar plexus is weak, that fire reduces to a lump of embers. It stops being effective as an incinerator. This is when we end up with indigestion, food allergies and sensitivities, stomachaches, poor absorption of nutrients, acid reflux, and heartburn. It also creates the conditions for unwelcome guests to proliferate.

My observation is that imbalances in gut bacteria, yeast, parasites, and so forth originate in tonal and vibrational imbalances in our system. This quickly becomes a vicious cycle: You start off with the tonal imbalance that creates the microbial imbalance, and then the microbial imbalance gets stronger and triggers a cascade of further tonal imbalances. Candida, for example, arises in the tonal valley of depression. Depression is often a consequence of "anger turned inward" that gets fed by sugar, and together, they put out your fire. We can't completely eliminate candida, because it naturally exists in the body, but what we can do is create a more resonant internal environment where the candida naturally falls into harmonious levels instead of reaching dissonant, detrimental levels.

Based on what I've seen in my work, a fundamental part of healing these imbalances (many of which are inherited, energenetic imbalances) is bringing our inner symphonies into balance, getting all the parts and pieces playing the right notes in the right way. Your gut is a symphony of microorganisms that are either living happily together and getting their groove on or they're having a hard time. I really believe that the gut microbiome can be rehabilitated, even without supplementation. It can be tonally rehabilitated by addressing the underlying emotional and mental patterns that are giving rise to the imbalance.

The sacral imbalances we discussed in the last chapter, most often related to the inner critic, suck the power away from our entire digestive tract, but especially the lower GI. The quivering of guilt and shame dampens the digestive fire and turns it into a whimper. I have yet to find a lower GI issue that wasn't emotional in nature. Crohn's, SIBO, ulcerative colitis, and IBS are all related to emotional suppression and disconnection, including in children. A child won't say, "I have anxiety." They'll say, "I have a stomachache. I don't feel good." Instead of identifying and expressing our emotions, we're creating this thing that we can give a name to. That continues in adulthood. We take on a stomachache to mask some complex emotion that we don't understand and we're not dealing with.

Here's one thing I recommend if you're struggling with digestive issues: Anytime you have a stomachache or some digestive discomfort, ask yourself what emotion is there. Go a little deeper: *Why is there a weakness in my system that's making it so that my gut isn't functioning properly?* The other thing to do is consciously direct more energy and voltage to your gut to help stoke the fire and get your digestion moving and shaking again. If I eat something that doesn't agree with me, instead of feeling gross and guilty and going into a story of victimhood around it, I just send more voltage to my stomach. I'll mobilize the troops and use the power of my intention to send some extra resources down to my gut to help out.

There's a kind of inner management that we can apply here. I owned a restaurant years ago, and when we got really slammed at lunchtime, I'd run around the whole restaurant picking up the slack wherever we were falling behind. If the dishwasher needed help, I'd get in there and wash dishes. If the sandwich bar was getting backed up, I'd get in there and help make sandwiches. Wherever things were starting to break down under load, I'd go in and shore them up. That's the same kind of attitude I apply with my body. *Something's falling behind; I'd better send in backup!* Instead of going into victim mode, you can just do a little consciousness hacking. All that's required is the recognition that you can consciously send more energy to wherever it's needed.

RESETTING THE ADRENALS

Another huge factor in digestion—as well as the health of the solar plexus and the system as a whole—is adrenal functioning.

The adrenals are two small endocrine glands, roughly the size of a walnut, that sit on top of your kidneys. Their job is to release hormones like adrenaline and cortisol into the bloodstream when your system is under stress, giving you the extra energy to help you deal with those stressors—that's the chemical perspective. From an electrical perspective, your kidney-adrenal complex is *very* electrically charged. When the adrenals release a surge of adrenaline, that's a flood of electricity and power into your system so that you can fight or run away. The adrenals are tiny, but they give off a huge amount of energy, with the adrenal field extending roughly three feet off the edge of the body. (Recent studies have also shown that our *bones* respond by releasing energy when we are under stress as well.)

The right and left adrenals have different personalities and different departments that they work with. The right adrenal, I've found, is connected with interpersonal and social stress. I call it the *office politics adrenal*. If your boss is a jerk or you're fighting with your spouse, your physical organism may not be under threat, but the emotional stress will activate the right adrenal. Even self-righteousness can get the right adrenal cranking. When out of balance, the right adrenal becomes a martyr. There's a sense that if it wasn't working overtime, then nothing would get done. It feels like it needs to run all the time just to keep the system going. If you have this kind of voice running in your mind, you've probably got that going in your right adrenal.

The left adrenal goes off when we're under physical threat. I call it the *saber-toothed tiger adrenal*. This is the classic fight-or-flight response. The "threat" to our physical safety may be current, from decades ago, or both. The history of the adrenal rhythm stays in the current adrenal rhythm, and it's informed by anything that's ever happened until we come along and reset it. If you were physically or even verbally abused when you were young, the left adrenal will go into overdrive. I've even seen the left adrenal go off in people who have a particularly vicious inner critic, which can be the embodied voice of the abusive parent (even one who isn't around anymore). If you have a bad habit of attacking yourself emotionally—or even physically hurting yourself by working too hard, not taking care of yourself (especially overexercising) and not getting enough rest—that can create a perception of physical threat in the system.

The adrenals, like every organ and system in the body, have their own rhythm. What I encounter consistently is an adrenal rhythm that runs too high and too fast, although sometimes it can also be sludgy or, in rare cases, go off-line altogether. Modern living can cause the adrenals to get stuck in the on position, leading to a wide variety of symptoms, including poor sleep, high stress reactivity, a short fuse, low thyroid, and impaired digestion (what alternative medicine has come to describe as *adrenal fatigue*). If you've been under too much stress for too long, it's almost like a toilet with a stuck handle that's running and running. When the adrenals have been going too fast for too long, they eventually burn out, and we end up in a state of exhaustion and depression.

It's very hard to feel like you have it together when your adrenals are falling apart. The adrenal imbalances I see are most often connected to a system that is chronically overworked and overburdened. We'll pile our plate up too high, we'll say *yes* when we mean *no*, we'll overschedule and overcommit because this old feeling of being in overdrive is just so familiar and comfortable. That rhythm can get set at birth. The way people respond to stress at the very beginning of life generally becomes the way they respond to stress through life. We start our lives in a too-fast adrenal rhythm, and then we keep creating circumstances that perpetuate it. If this goes on for long enough, we eventually shift from the hyped-up overdrive into exhaustion and depletion.

This is another area that is largely culturally influenced. There's a huge amount of social pressure for us to be on and going all the time, and it destroys the adrenals. Back when I was in prep school, we had classes, activities, and sports from 8:00 a.m. to 5:00 p.m. every day, plus three hours of homework every night and games on the weekends. Today, the overscheduling of children starts in preschool. Children's playtime has been continuously declining since the 1970s alongside a sharp rise in depression and anxiety disorders in early childhood. This kind of model engenders a deep pattern of overdoing that throws off the basic rhythm of our system.

We pay the price of habitually pushing through it not only in our well-being in the present moment but in years shaved off our lives. What we're doing to our kids when we deprive them of play and rest and free time is not healthy. To what end are we putting our kids, and ourselves, through this level of stress?

We need to question on a deep level what is healthy and appropriate for us in our lives beyond what our culture and upbringing have instilled in us. What is your body telling you? I like to think of my body as my horse. If your horse is tired and needs to rest, but instead you whip the horse to make it keep going, your horse is going to die much sooner than it would if you had honored and respected it as a natural organism. When you look at your body as the horse that's carrying you through this life, you start to reconsider: Do you really want to be whipping that horse and forcing it to go, go, go? That's when you start running on adrenaline, because you don't have any natural energy left. When you're in this mode, your whole system gets out of whack eventually. Your adrenals burn out. You become more susceptible to food allergies. Your immunity weakens, and you get sick all the time. Your digestive fire becomes a pile of embers, and you're not pulling out the nutrients from your food. You lose your libido.

People often seek to treat adrenal fatigue with diet and supplements, but I've found that unless the underlying *rhythm* of the adrenals is adjusted, this offers only a Band-Aid solution. Sound can be used like an adaptogen for the adrenals. The body uses the coherent rhythm introduced into the field to recognize its own lack of rhythm and to autocorrect. A while back, I developed a technique called the *adrenal reset,* where we introduce a tuning fork at the edge of the field off either side of the solar plexus and slowly work in toward the midline of the body with our attention on the kidney/adrenal system, listening to the record of that rhythm from conception on. As the tuning fork moves through this record, it acts as a metronome, helping the body recalibrate the adrenals back to a healthy rhythm. Coupled with the intention to bring the adrenals into greater harmony, I've found that this method can be truly life-changing for people. Once their inner vibes of stress change, their outer lives reconfigure to reflect that. I have a recorded adrenal reset session available in the Biofield Tuning online store for folks who are interested in trying this approach. You can also make use of a single tuning fork that you hold on or over your kidneys, using it like a stethoscope to monitor and feel into the rhythm. Allow that conversation of incoherent versus coherent rhythms to take place until a greater sense of harmony is sensed.

Beyond sound and adequate rest, one of the best healing tonics for the adrenals—and the solar plexus as a whole—is *play*. We need to give ourselves permission to not be so goal-oriented and to just kick up our heels every once in a while. Under the exhaustion and anger and martyrdom, there's an inherent brightness and joyfulness in the solar plexus that wants to sing and dance. What thrills you? For me, it's exploring. I love adventures. Whenever I have the chance, I take my husband off driving around country roads we've never been on before because that's what makes me happy. Exploring the biofield has been so thrilling because it's this whole territory that's been hidden in plain view. Every single session is an adventure because you never know what you are going to encounter, and that makes me incredibly happy.

One of the big reasons why we want to get healthier, have more money, and be more successful is to feel free—and to feel free is to have more fun. Ask yourself: *If I'm not feeling angry or powerless, can I be playful?* As we start to heal ourselves, we are naturally inclined to what makes us happy. To play, to be creative through music and art, to freely experience the joyful parts of life. And through that playfulness, we are led to a greater sense of gratitude, joy, and connection to others and all of life— which lifts us up to the energy of the heart.

13

HEART: Opening to Love

Your heart is the electromagnetic motor for your whole system. Not only does it keep you alive by pumping oxygenated blood throughout your body, it's also constantly receiving and transmitting electrical currents to and from your environment and throughout your system. The electromagnetic field of the heart is the most powerful field produced by the body, extending out several feet in each direction. It informs every cell of your being and can be detected at any point on the surface of the body.

Simply put, the heart is our electrical connection to life. We're a part of our electromagnetic environment, and the ambient electricity surrounding us at every moment is what keeps us alive. You've learned that you're not just breathing in oxygen from the air; you're also breathing in plasma, charged particles, light, and movement. Your heart pumps that energy throughout your veins, into all your organs, tissues, and bones and throughout the plasma bubble that is your human biofield. It's this energy that's keeping us alive. Think about it: If someone's heart stops, we apply *electricity* to jump-start it.

In the biofield anatomy, the heart center governs the physical heart and circulatory system, the arms, shoulders, and hands, and also the lungs and diaphragm. It holds the expression of giving and receiving love but can also harbor difficult-to-feel emotions like hate, resentment, grief, sadness, depression, and despair. Physically, imbalances in the heart chakra can manifest as shallow breathing, asthma, shoulder, arm, or hand pain, upper back pain, poor posture, and any number of cardiovascular conditions. The harmonious expression of the heart is reflected in the color green, the vowel sound "ahh," and the seed syllable "YAM."

Heart disease is the number-one killer in the United States. We talk about the role of diet and smoking and saturated fat in heart health, but I rarely hear anyone discussing the *emotions* that inform the heart, beyond the somewhat vague label of "stress." My observation from an electrical perspective is that heart disease is the body's response to unmanageable emotions. When we carry emotional burdens for too long, the physical heart gets strained. The heart is strongly impacted by grief, despair, sadness, and hate, and a backlog of these emotions will impair its physical functioning. When we harden our squishy, tender hearts to keep out tough emotions, we arrest that flow of life and electricity that's pumping through the heart at every moment. My experience is that people have heart attacks when their electrical relationship with life has been severed by pushing away themselves, other people, and life itself.

In the file drawers to the sides of the heart center, particularly around the left and right shoulders, we find information and emotions related to unhealthy or imbalanced expressions of love as well as the lack or loss of love. The left side of the heart holds unprocessed sadness, depression, and grief, often passed down through generational and ancestral channels. If a person suffers from depression in particular, there will be a lot of stuck energy here. On the right side of the heart, I find imbalances related to over-accommodating and over-caretaking, putting others' needs before our own, saying *yes* when we mean *no,* and the feeling of resentment. Directly over the physical heart is where we encounter the emotion of hate. This is a tough one that many of us (especially nice, spiritual folks) don't want to admit that we feel. Something I regularly observe is how people suppress their hate and self-loathing and then end up projecting it onto others.

This is pretty heavy-duty stuff. There's a *lot* going on in the heart, which is a part of why I prefer the solar plexus as a place to rest my awareness. Yes, there is love and compassion, but we have to wade through all these very charged emotions to get there. When your consciousness is centered in your core, it's easier to keep your heart open. With a strong sense of self and strong boundaries in place, we're able to love and care for others in a way that honors the needs of our own organism.

RESTING IN LOVE AND GRATITUDE

When the heart center is open and coherent, we are able to easily and spontaneously feel love toward ourselves, other people, and all of life. I don't just mean saying, "I love you"—I mean *really* feeling the force of love swell up from deep inside you. Love of self. Love of family. Love of friends. Love of nature. Love of the universe. We are able to rest in love, throughout our whole beings, which is really the most energy-efficient place to hang out.

A friend of mine always says, "If it's a cliché, it must be true." It's true that love is the most healing force on the planet. I truly believe that love conquers all. It's the sun that always rises. Some spiritual philosophies say that everything that isn't love is fear, and I tend to agree. I've concluded that everything is love, and anything that isn't love is just static or distortion. Underneath the noise of the pain body, it's all just love.

But let's expand our perception of love for a moment. We've been conditioned to think of love in terms of romance and sex and heterosexual dyads and fairy-tale happy endings. But love is so much more than that. Nature unfolds in this perfect geometry, and that perfection is what we call goodness, truth, beauty, love. It's all the same thing. It all points to the sweet spot in the signal, the perfect sine wave. When you're in that vibration, when you're hanging out on a summer day and everything's peachy, that's love. Nature lives in that sweet spot. Everyone wants that, not just hippies and hopeless romantics.

As you make your way through this chapter, I invite you to examine your own beliefs about love. Is there cynicism? Is there hurt? Fear? A sense of lack? Honor whatever beliefs are there while inviting the possibility of a more expanded perspective. You don't have to change or get rid of any limiting beliefs that might be there, but maybe you can also entertain the idea of love winning or the idea that love has already won.

The healing power of love is a biological reality. When you open your heart to love, you create more coherence in your system and in your life. Among its many key functions, your heart is also the driving rhythm of your body. It sets the tone for everything else. I think of it as the mother in the family: *If Mama ain't happy, ain't nobody happy.* When the heart is in a coherent state, it beats in a rhythmic and consistent manner. Researchers at the HeartMath Institute have studied this phenomenon extensively, tracking heart rate variability patterns while people were feeling positive emotions like love, gratitude, and joy. They've observed that under the influence of positive emotions, the heart's rhythm became more consistent and orderly. The rhythm of heart rate variability generated by these coherent emotions created a perfect sine wave.

The best way to get the heart into a coherent state is by consciously feeling love and gratitude. Remember that we're all actors and actresses, and we have the ability to conjure up these emotions in our beings. Gratitude is a good place to start, because it's so readily available. No matter what's going on in our lives, there's so much that we can be grateful for. In his excellent book *Happy Money,* Ken Honda talks about saying thank you ten thousand times a day. Honda explains that he first received this advice from a little old Japanese man, so it was actually, *"Arigato! Arigato! Arigato!"* We can be grateful for anything and everything. I'm so grateful I can get out of bed. I'm so grateful for this warm shower. I'm grateful for my coffee. Throughout my day, I stop and think to myself, *Arigato! Arigato!*

There is an actual energetic impact to the experience of gratitude. My good friend Dr. Paul Mills has done a number of studies measuring how gratitude improves your health and well-being, and the data is compelling. Gratitude immediately anchors you back into your heart, back in your center, calling your energy back to you and making it available for use. It also gives you the perspective to ask if you really need to do or have more than you're currently doing or having. Are you coming from a place of contentment or a place of lack? A moment of gratitude will make it clear.

I recently had a very powerful experience of gratitude. It was my fiftieth birthday, and fate had arranged itself so that was the day we were launching the Tuners Without Borders program at Boys' Town school in Trench Town, Jamaica, right across the street from where Bob Marley lived as a youth. So many things conspired on that day, including receiving a generous donation from Tony Robbins toward our efforts, and it all added up to create one of the most amazing experiences I have ever had. I was walking down the hallway of the hotel in Kingston and reflecting on this incredible day, and I was feeling so much gratitude for the powers that be that I suddenly felt my biofield expand, almost as if it were reaching out to God and being reached out to by God in this sort of explosive, ecstatic, transcendent experience. It was truly one of the most extraordinary visceral experiences I have ever had. It was as if my gratitude became so big that it actually exploded out of me. After it settled, I thought of Paul. If anyone would understand what had happened to me, he would. When I described my experience, I told him that *transcendence* was the best word I could come up with, and he told me that it actually is a recognized thing—and it's actually called transcendence!

Don't underestimate the ability of a practice of gratitude to shift things up for you. It is a very powerful force!

LETTING DOWN THE HEART SHIELD

Healing the heart is a process of softening and opening, like a peony in bloom. Peonies start off as these tiny golf balls and then explode into a universe of multidimensional beauty. I've seen that when the heart softens, feelings of separation and loneliness give way to an expansive sense of warmth and connectivity. Strained relationships naturally begin to heal. The physical heart becomes squishy and soft again, and the emotional heart is open and tender and warm. We return to a state of what's known in Tibetan Buddhism as *tsewa*, the innate tenderness of heart that is an essential quality of enlightenment.

There is a common structure that I encounter called the *heart shield*. That shield gets put up when we're in a position, often early in life, in which we really have no choice but to protect our tender hearts from difficult characters or situations. It's understandable, as the emotions that preceded the shutdown were really hard to take. If you grew up in a home that was abusive or unpredictable, you learn to shut down to protect yourself. If you had a Jekyll-and-Hyde parent who gave love and then withdrew it, that's going to really confuse your system. After a while of that back-and-forth, you start to put up a false front because you can't handle getting hurt anymore.

We put up the heart shield to cope with the unmanageable situation, and then we keep it up as a way to protect ourselves from having to feel into the hurt that the heart is holding. What happens over time is that the heart hardens, leading to stiffening arteries, heart disease, and heart attacks.

Once we start to gently process and release the emotions residing in the heart, once we allow ourselves to feel the hurt, grief, and sadness that's there, the heart doesn't need to harden to keep them out anymore. Take some time to explore and investigate your heart history. Have you been hard-hearted toward yourself or anyone else? Where have you shut down your heart? Did you see this in either one of your parents?

Feel into what's going on in your heart. When you bring your awareness there, can you feel any areas that have become tight or stiffened? Use your active imagination to explore your heart and any shielding that might be there. When we bring any thought form or energetic structure into the light of awareness, it naturally starts to dissolve that structure. Direct your breath there to open up space. Allow that soft, youthful heart to come back into expression, knowing (or at least being open to the possibility) that it's safe for the heart to be open.

We put on our armor for good reason, but at some point, we have to ask ourselves if we still need to move through the world from a defended place. Very slowly and gently, we want to begin to let down our defenses and climb out of our shells. We want to start trusting that it's safe to allow our hearts to be open and vulnerable. One of our Biofield Tuning instructors, Lori Rhoades (who has a wonderful way with words), talks about availability versus vulnerability. If the idea of vulnerability feels scary to you, flip the script and ask yourself if you can be *available*. They're really the same thing, but availability can feel a little safer, and we need to support the heart in feeling safe. Instead of feeling fearful and disempowered in your vulnerability, you can become empowered in your availability: showing up, fully present, petals open.

RIGHT SIDE: OVER-GIVING, SAYING *YES* WHEN WE MEAN *NO*

The yang imbalances of the right side of the heart occur when we give to others at the expense of our own well-being. It's over-caretaking and over-accommodating. I call the right shoulder the *nice girl* or *yes-man shoulder*. The tendency to say *yes* when we mean *no* is a huge pattern here. Over time, it creates dissonance in the entire heart region and blocks the natural flow of giving and receiving. These patterns are often driven by a deep-rooted fear of being cast out of the tribe. That fear of what other people think gets programmed into the right arm. We end up sacrificing ourselves and overdoing for others because we want to be loved and accepted, and we're afraid of being rejected and isolated if we don't.

There are a few particular personality types that I tend to encounter in this zone. The big one is the helper personality: They are often healers, caregivers, and those who work in service professions or run nonprofit organizations. Another is the oldest child, who grew up being expected to caretake for younger siblings. They end up in roles where they're the ones who are always in charge and taking care of everyone else, and they feel a sense of responsibility for everything. Then there's the empath, who feels the emotions of others on a deep level and consciously or unconsciously takes on a responsibility for relieving their suffering. Yet another is the child who was forced to become the parent, due to their own parent not being able to fulfill that role for whatever reason.

Right heart and shoulder issues (as well as solar plexus imbalances) occur frequently in people who had enmeshed or codependent relation-ships with their parents. This happens with women especially, and it is one of the most difficult things you can go through as a child. It strips away our sense of play and lightness. There's no space for that process of discovery of who we are and what makes us happy, and a big part of ourselves gets stunted. Very often, we end up repeating an old pattern of invalidating our own emotions and sacrificing ourselves to please others.

I have a girlfriend who owns a massage school, has a busy massage practice, and teaches at three different colleges. She's also a single mom. Not that long ago, she called me and said, "Hey, Eileen, I got an injury. Guess where it is?" I said, "It's in your right shoulder, isn't it?" "Yup," she responded. She fell while she was hiking, and it's no surprise to me that this is where she landed. If your energy is out of balance in a certain area, you've got a weakness and vulnerability in that part of your physical anatomy. If you're ever experiencing right shoulder pain, you have to ask yourself, *How am I overextending myself? How am I compromising the physical well-being of my body?* Or think back to any times in your life that you in-jured this shoulder. What was going on then?

When we dishonor ourselves to try to honor other people, it's not a win-win. It's not healthy or right. It's bad for our physical hearts and our emo-tional well-being. Our cultural notions of "politeness" are a part of the problem. Beyond politeness, many of us have also fallen prey to the cul-tural ideal of service above self. We're conditioned to believe that looking after our own wants and needs is selfish. But the reality is this: *Serving to the detriment of our own health and well-being is not noble.* Of course, there are times we find ourselves in positions where we really don't have any choice about putting aside our own goals and desires to attend to the needs of others. There was a time in my life when I was taking care of my father in his last year of life. My mom, who had been taking care of him, had passed away. At the time, I also had a newborn baby who didn't sleep, and I was trying to run two businesses. I had no choice about being a care-taker. I had to take care of my dad, my son, and my businesses, and at that time, I was incapable of establishing clear boundaries and taking care of myself—as a result I ended up strung out and resentful!

When we habitually put others over self, resentment is the result. It builds and settles on and around the right shoulder, and then it comes out in passive-aggressive behavior or distance in relationships or getting to a point where we just snap and can't be around that person anymore. You end up blaming and punishing the person that you're saying yes to. That's misplaced, because you're the one putting yourself in that position. Step back and ask yourself if you have a choice instead of defaulting into that habitual role. Is this a place where you can say no, set a boundary, take care of yourself first? When you first start saying no, you may feel guilty, but you'll get through that stage, and you'll ultimately find the proper balance of energetic output and input. Saying no when appropriate is better for you, it's better for them, and ultimately, it preserves and strengthens your relationships. There's always a peaceful path, you just have to look for it.

Even as a caretaker, you have to put on your own oxygen mask first. We now have a generation that's caretaking for children with autism and parents with Alzheimer's. If you're caretaking two generations and you have a full-time job, how are you going to deal with that? You've got to take care of your own organism. You've got to raise your voltage. You have to find it in yourself to take good care of yourself despite everyone else's needs. You've got to find moments in the day when you can catch the updraft. Otherwise, you're not going to make it. And we need you to make it! We're in a time in our collective human experience when there's a lot of need all around us. We need superheroes.

If you're stuck between your aging parents and your children, or some other complex caregiver arrangement, there's a certain patience that is called for. You can't just drop everything to go follow your bliss. But you can choose, in small places here and there, to raise your voltage and increase your capacity to do what you need to do for others *and* for yourself.

Here's another thing to keep in mind: While we don't have a choice about some relationships—family in particular—we *do* have a choice about others. Part of good energy management is people management. Start becoming conscious of whom you're spending time with and how it's impacting your energy. Energy is electromagnetic, and it flows from areas of greater concentration to areas of lesser concentration. Sometimes we can't even help it that when we're hanging out with someone, we've just flowed our energies into them. We all know people who are so incapable of meeting their own needs that when you're with them, they suck the life out of you. Engaging with this kind of person is not a give-and-take. It's all needy needy. Again, we don't always have a choice, especially if we're caretakers. But whenever possible, we're much better off keeping the company of people who are like those Himalayan salt lamps—they spread extra charge to whomever they are with without depleting themselves. They make you light up and feel good. Spend more time with these types of folks, and strive to be one yourself. Hang out with electron donors, not electron stealers. And aim to be one yourself!

LEFT SIDE: SADNESS, DEPRESSION, GRIEF, AND LOSS

The left side of the heart was the very first area I identified in the biofield anatomy, when I realized that I kept finding sad stories in this area. Sadness is very easy to recognize with the forks because it sounds so much like sad music. There's no mistaking it.

We harbor a lot of old pain and hurt here, almost always connected to some lack or loss of love. We hold the energy of sadness around the loss of loved ones; experiences of neglect, abuse, abandonment, and betrayal; the end of relationships, jobs, dreams, or anything else that we hold dear in our hearts. I've sifted through a lot of different expressions of sadness in this zone, including grief, loss, depression, betrayal, disappointment, loneliness, melancholy, and abandonment. There's a lot of pain in here for all of us and our families and our ancestors, and we want to honor that. It's very much a part of the human story. It's the first noble truth of Buddhism: *Life is suffering.* It is impossible to make your way through a human life without hurt, loss, and pain.

This is another area with a lot of ancestral influence. If your parents, particularly your mother, carried a lot of sadness, a piece of that sadness is in you. In one of my practitioner trainings, I acted as the demonstration body for a segment that was focused on working with the shoulders. My co-teacher thought it would be easy and straightforward to work on me because I've had so much of this work done. But as she started on the outer edge of the field around the left side of my heart center, she almost immediately hit a patch of turbulence. What came in was my grandmother's energy, and it was unmistakably sad. The entire class could feel it, and even more interesting was that most of the class also had the immediate sense that it was an imprint from my mother's mother. It got even stronger as we hit the ancestral river. I had done what had sometimes felt like endless work processing my own backlog of sadness, as well as my mother's, and what do you know—here was yet another layer of the same pattern encoded in my DNA. So she got to work healing this grandmother energy, and all of a sudden, I felt this deep knot untie in my upper left shoulder blade. I went to see my massage therapist that night, and she asked me, "Why do your shoulders feel so different?" This knot that had been there for God knows how long just dissolved.

A nice visualization is to hold your mother and your mother's mother, then your entire maternal lineage, in your heart. Think about the degree of coherence versus incoherence that they may have had in their lives. Were they able to freely feel love, joy, and gratitude? Know that you can heal your parents and offspring through the work you do on yourself.

Much of the noise here is also related to not getting the love that we needed in childhood, including feelings of abandonment in people who were adopted or among those who were born premature and put in incubators. One time I worked on a friend who I didn't realize when I started the session had been an incubator baby for the first month of her life. As I was combing through the left side of her heart, I encountered what felt like a barrier between her and her mother. It felt like a glass wall. When I told her this, she told me the incubator story and that this feeling of glass between her and her mother had followed her for her whole life. She never felt like she could really connect with her mother, and she held on to a huge amount of sadness and frustration as a result. This sense of abandonment even shows up in babies who were taken away from their mothers by doctors or nurses immediately after they're born, which is a very common practice. Being separated from our mothers right after birth creates this sense of, *Where's my mom? Why am I not being touched and held and nursed?*

If you weren't loved as a child in the way that you wanted and needed to be, take a moment to send some love back to your infant self. Hold your inner child in your arms and just send him or her love. Tell your inner child whatever it was that you needed to hear. *You're going to make it through. You are loved. You are worthy.*

Remember that the nature of the universe is love. Anything that's not love is just noise in the signal. When you tell the story of "I'm not lovable," you're just energizing the noise. The heart is exquisitely tender, and for those of us who are sensitive, it's even tenderer. It reacts to both internal and external threats by throwing up the shield. See if you can speak to your tender heart with the sweet voice of kindness rather than the growl of the inner critic.

THE WORLD PAIN SPOT

Several years into my process of mapping the biofield, I made a new discovery the week that Robin Williams died by suicide. In nearly everyone who came in for a tuning that week, I noticed a bunch of stuck energy around the left armpit. As I listened into the tonal quality of that zone, I realized that the field was being energized by feelings of pain about the human condition and the state of the world.

There was so much collective sadness, shock, and disillusionment around the loss of Robin Williams. He had been one of the most beloved performers of his generation. People grew up watching him. So many of us felt like we knew him. There was a shared sense of shock and sadness that someone who made us laugh so much could be in enough pain to take his own life.

I came to think of this spot in the biofield anatomy as the *world pain zone*. Since then, I've noticed activation in that spot in a great many people— more and more so in recent years. The events that make us feel the suffering of the world can be intense and emotionally overwhelming for us. We're all exposed to other people's suffering, and we feel it deeply. Some folks just pour energy out of this spot if they are in the habit of bemoaning the state of the world and feeling sad and powerless about it.

The left armpit is the "pit of despair," so to speak. There's no end to things to feel bad about here. We are witnessing the sixth mass extinction right before our eyes. The planet is awash in plastic and pollution, refugees and refuse, injustice and inequality. We could sit and cry all day for what's going on in the world—for every species we're losing, for every waterway that's polluted, for every human being that's being denied their basic freedom, dignity, and survival needs.

That's an easy place to go to, but what good does it do to sit and cry all day? If you feel sad about the pollution of water (as I often do), go pick up trash next to your river. Make a twenty-dollar donation to an environmental organization that you trust. Do something. Go ahead and cry about it, but then see what can be done.

It's okay to have moments of despair. We don't want to deny this world pain. It's real. There's loss, grief, sadness, and hurt that needs to be acknowledged and honored. And yet we have to keep walking this tightrope as we move along our life path on planet Earth at this pivotal time in history. The path forward is narrow, and it's not easy to stay on track. It is very easy to fall off into world pain and just cry for hours. If that's what you need to do right now, then I invite you to honor that. But if you're making a habit of it, you have to ask yourself whether it's helping. If you're telling yourself a story of victimhood and powerlessness, it is certainly not helping. If you're sinking over there in the left-hand ditch, you're not improving the situation for yourself or anyone else.

When we allow ourselves to get stuck in world pain, we're also just pouring more incoherent vibes into the whole mess. I'm not saying you shouldn't feel world pain. I feel it every day, and I am easily brought to tears over whatever tragedy crosses the path of my awareness, but I don't stay there. That's because I also easily feel gratitude and amazement and wonder and even grace. The world is full of pain and suffering and injustice, but it is also still full of music and miracles, opportunities for joy and love and wonder, reasons to be grateful and amazed. It's not *either-or*, it's *both-and:* pain and beauty, suffering and joy, hatred and love, destruction and rebirth.

Start to tune in to what happens in your energy field when you go into world pain. Notice how the energy of your heart shifts to the left and sinks in there. See if you can open your heart wider to hold the pain and grief alongside gratitude and curiosity. Try shifting your inner energetic posture from your left armpit to the center of your chest. Shift your awareness from sadness and heaviness to gratitude and love.

In the study of sound, there's something called *cymatics,* which describes the effect that sound waves and vibration have on matter. The practice goes back at least one thousand years to African tribes that would sprinkle grains on the skin of drums and play different sounds to create patterns in the grain, which were then used for prophecies. If you watch a video of cymatics (I highly recommend you go find one on YouTube), you'll see that when the frequency changes, the old pattern of matter (whether it's sand or metal filings or anything else) breaks down as a new pattern simultaneously emerges. There's chaos and order, entropy and syntropy, taking place at the same time. Even as things are seemingly going into the toilet in our country and across the globe, a potentially beautiful new order is arising. I believe we're witnessing a "turning of the ages." It can feel pretty unpleasant in the chaos, but that chaos is necessary for the new structure to arise. As that's happening all around us, we have a choice where we place our attention. We can put our attention on what's collapsing, or we can focus on what's coming into being. It's when we're looking at all the entropy in the world and panicking that we start falling off our path.

Ask yourself: *Where is the syntropy right now?* Wherever there's powerful entropy, there's going to be powerful syntropy. We can allow ourselves to be pulled into the descending current, or we can choose to follow the updraft. Whatever we put our focus on expands. If you focus solely on what's falling apart, that will be your experience. You can identify with that and freak out, or you can ask yourself, *Hmm, what new order is arising, and how can I be a part of that? How can I separate from the fear of the chaos and the dissolution and move into a place where I'm aligning with what's arising?*

Let's reframe it: *If some things are going down and other things are coming up, I'm going to go over there and be part of the coming-up.* This is a wild time to be alive! It really is. It can feel really rough, but the healthier you are, you can reframe it and ask what role you have to play at this pivotal time in history.

HEALING HATE

At the center of the chaos we're seeing in the world right now is a collective release of anger and hate. We're getting rid of this backlog of emotions not only for ourselves but for previous generations who weren't able to express themselves, and that's a good thing. But it also asks us to bring more consciousness to hate so that we can manage it without causing harm to ourselves and others. The bottom line is that regularly engaging in conscious or subconscious hate is definitely not a healthy or voltage-raising practice!

Hate is a difficult emotion for many reasons. It's something we don't like to talk about, let alone *feel*. Brené Brown has done a great job of getting people to recognize and talk about shame, but nobody likes to talk about hate. Growing up, we're told that "hate is a strong word." We shouldn't speak it, and we shouldn't feel it. We're programmed with an abstinence-only, "just say no" approach to hate. As a result, we turn a valid emotion that arises from natural bodily responses into something that's denied and turned inward. Instead of seeking to understand *why* we hate something and working to correct that, we're simply told to suppress it.

There are two camps when it comes to hate: people who suppress their hate and turn it inward, and those who externalize it with bigotry, aggression, hate speech, and hate crimes. Generally, the people who internalize their hate then end up hating the haters. They hate Trump, they hate white supremacists, they hate racists and homophobes and misogynists. We end up in a situation where hate is circulating all around. And just about everybody seems to carry around some degree of self-hatred.

We have to acknowledge and accept that even nice, good, spiritual people experience hate, and that's okay. Hate is a valid emotion. It's not a bad thing to feel hate, but we want to admit it. Be honest with yourself: *What do you hate?* Give yourself permission to feel hate if it's arising. Be curious about it. Most often, hate arises when we feel hurt, scared, angry, and powerless. It is a valid reaction to an unhealthy or painful situation. Allow it legitimacy. Ask yourself if you can forgive and allow the energy to move through your heart in a natural way so that you can be open to feeling more love and compassion.

When I moved to Burlington, Vermont, I found myself driving around bicyclists all the time. I'd never lived anywhere that I had to deal with that before. In a very short amount of time, I found myself starting to hate bicyclists. I was taken aback, in fact, by the amount of hatred I felt toward them. It was really weird to be feeling so much hate! I declared my hatred of bicyclists to several of my friends, some of whom were offended and taken aback by it. I decided that I preferred not to continue getting all charged up with hate, so I decided to take a look at where it was coming from and really try to understand it.

What I discovered was that there were a few different emotions in the mix. For one, I was feeling powerless because I had very little control over the situation. The bicyclists seemed to do whatever they wanted, and I couldn't predict their behavior. There was also fear that I was going to hurt one of them or that they were going to hurt me, as well as a sense of hurt at what I perceived as their lack of sensitivity and concern for the safety of others. So there I was feeling afraid and powerless and hurt, and I was also a little angry about the whole situation.

More often than not, hate is a tangled knot with a lot of pieces. For the sake of our own health, we want to untangle these strands so that we can release the charge from our bodies. As soon as I was able to break it down and address each one of those feelings individually, the charge began to lift on its own. I was able to say to myself, *This is what's going on in my environment. How can I learn to live with it?* I realized that I had to adapt and overcome instead of getting trapped in this web of emotions that wasn't good for my body or for the people around me.

If you're distressed about the hate going on around you, know that you can change the signal. Instead of tuning in to all the fear and hate around us, we can tune in to the love that's being broadcast from the hearts of good people. For all the terrible things that humanity does, there is an equal if not greater amount of kindness, compassion, love, and generosity. There are so many hearts working toward love, coherence, and freedom from fear. We can find solidarity here.

There's a lot of love being broadcast through the aether! The coherent heart signal is always there, we just have to tune in to it.

CONSCIOUSLY RECEIVING LOVE AND GRATITUDE

Through the back of the heart chakra, we receive love and gratitude. So many of us have been programmed, because we don't feel worthy, to not allow ourselves to receive positive attention. We push love away because we don't think we deserve to let it in. If someone pays us a compliment, we shut it down. We don't really accept loving attention from others. Over the years, people have given me a lot of gratitude for helping them to feel better. Initially, it made me uncomfortable, and it took some very conscious heart opening for me to allow myself to receive that.

Love and appreciation are a currency, and when someone offers them to you, you'd be wise to soak them up like a sponge. Think of them as electrons being donated. You can let those electrons energize your heart and your whole being.

We lose so much when we can't receive: What that person is trying to give you is a form of energy, and we need that electricity to replenish our own battery reserves. There are so many places we can receive love from! Are you letting the universe love you? Are you letting the sunlight love you? We're bathing in a sea of love. It's all around us. Think about all the people who are praying and chanting and sending love, all the holy people and Reiki practitioners and meditators who are sending love all the time. There are so many people out there sending out prayers, love, and healing at every moment. Nature itself is giving us the codes to be fully healed all the time.

I was hiking not that long ago, and my left knee started to go south.

As I was coming down the mountain, it was really giving me a hard time. So I stood in front of this beautiful beech tree and I just let it love and heal me, and it did, and somewhat amazingly, I was able to walk down the rest of the trail with no pain. It didn't even hurt at all the next day. Love is all around you. Love is healing you all the time. It's a great mind hack to just be able to go into that. Let that love in. Let a flower or a tree or a cool breeze just love you up.

THROAT: The Resonance of Truth

As a sound therapist, writer, and singer, I have a particular affinity for the throat chakra. Governing the mouth, jaw, ears, and faculty of hearing, in addition to the physical throat and thyroid gland, the throat is our center of creative expression and communication. It is through our throat that we create and hear sound; and it's also in the throat center that we come into resonance with the truth of our beings.

I often say that the throat is the most powerful energy center that I work on. That is because it is through our *word* that we create our lives. It's difficult to overestimate the power of the word, for it is the quality of our words that determines the quality of our lives. As we speak, so we create.

How are you using the creative power of your word? What unbeneficial mantras are you repeating over and over and thus continually creating, unwittingly? It is my observation that what comes *out* of our mouths, rather than what we put into them, plays a far greater role in determining our health and happiness. We tend to pay a lot of attention to what we're eating and comparatively less to what we're saying. If you're eating cleanly but you're constantly saying to yourself and others, *I have Hashimoto's. I'm sick. I'm not healthy. My body is failing on me,* then you are missing the point of how creative your word is.

It is astounding what you can learn from paying close attention to what people say and the tones of their voices while they're saying it. I'm a syntax nut, particularly when it comes to a person's declarative statements about who they are and what's going on in their life. If someone says *I am* or *I have* in reference to something that they'd prefer not to be or have, I will be ruthless in jumping right on them. I am strong in my insistence on the creative power of the word.

But it's not just the words coming out of your mouth—it's the words in your head. Thoughts are phenomenally creative. We are continually creating with what we think, believe, and say. In the Hindu tradition, there are tales of wish-fulfilling divine trees called *kalpatarus,* which are just a metaphor for the mind. We have thoughts, and sooner or later, those thoughts are fulfilled. This is the true meaning of "Be careful what you wish for."

The biofield around the throat area holds the history of our communication or lack thereof. The impulse to express something is an electromagnetic event, and if it is suppressed, it accumulates and builds up in the system, creating static and inflammation. "Better out than in!" is one of the profound truths I've seen in this work.

In the biofield anatomy, the left side of the throat relates to that which we don't say and express. It holds the imprint of the words and emotions we swallow (there tends to be a lot of inherited trauma here from generations of stifled expression). On the right, we find information related to speaking but not being heard. Imbalances on either side of the throat can result in thyroid issues as well as tightness of breath (a kind of bottleneck effect) and neck and jaw tension. We want to bring both sides of the throat chakra into alignment, centered above the heart, so that we can more easily commit to speaking and living our truths. When the throat is in balance, we communicate clearly and we are heard by others, we use the power of language to create and manifest that which we desire. To connect with the healthy resonance of the throat, you can visualize the color blue, hum or tone the vowel sound "eye," and repeat the seed syllable "HAM."

When we reach the fifth energy center, we also start to tap into the power of sound through the vehicle of our voices. What does your voice sound like? Are you speaking in neutral mid-tones? Is your voice high and pinched, or low and muffled? Every time you speak, it's like sound therapy for your body, so you want to start paying attention to your tone of voice. Move it around! Shake it up! Do high tones and low tones. Be expressive. Practice using your voice in a more varied way so that you're really moving energy through that whole throat center.

You can sing. You can repeat mantras. You can hum. Sound healer Jonathan Goldman wrote a whole book on the health benefits of humming—give it a try! Or try toning the vowel sounds or seed mantras of each center. There's a simple toning exercise I use to help shake up old patterns of tonality and support greater resonance: Visualize your throat chakra as whatever beautiful shade of blue you like, and then vocalize several rounds of *ahhhhhhhhh,* breathing in deep and then extending the *ahhh* tone on the exhale for as long as you can.

Your voice is a built-in sound healing tool. Singing has been scientifically proven to reduce stress hormone levels and increase levels of the oxytocin (the love hormone) and feel-good endorphins. When we sing or chant, our breathing slows down, which calms the nervous system and quiets down the body's stress response. The bones and the fluid in the body conducts sound, and when we use our voices, waves of sound travel through the system, releasing tension and relaxing the nervous system. Try directing the sound of your voice into different organs, joints or any part of your body that feels tense to give it a little "sound massage"—it really works!

When the back of the throat center is open, it brings in inspiration from the deepest part of our beings, clearing a pathway for our inner wisdom and artistry to emerge. A few years ago, I was working on one woman's throat and asking her if she was a writer. "No," she said. "Why?" I kept listening to the tone of the forks in her field. "It really seems to me like you're a writer." When I saw her again for the first time a couple of years later, she had written a whole children's book series. She told me that she started it after she left that appointment. It was as if the sound pulled out the cork from the back of her throat and let the inspiration flow. The back of the throat opens up our ability to receive inspiration so that we can communicate it. What is the universe wanting you to say? What is your soul asking you to communicate? Can you soften and open that portal so that information can flow more freely?

The throat chakra also encompasses the mouth and our relationship to pleasure in the mouth. Through our mouths, we express who we are to the world, and we also take in the world around us, breathing in oxygen and life force. Through our mouths, we enjoy food and the sensual pleasures of taste. The mouth is a pleasure center! It has a sensuality that is very much connected to the sacral chakra. Through both of these centers, we are able to give and receive pleasure: to share intimacy, to speak beauty, to make beautiful sounds. But instead of experiencing pleasure with our mouths, so many of us engage in mindless consumption. The ability to sit and savor food without guilt, to just eat with pleasure and gratitude and blessings, is a key to a healthy throat chakra.

SPEAK YOUR TRUTH: THE SECRET TO THYROID HEALTH (AND HIGH VOLTAGE)

One of the most profound lessons for me in all my years of Biofield Tuning has been seeing how many people don't speak their truths. We do this in all kinds of ways. We repress our emotions until we stuff and blow, we say what others want to hear and not what we really feel, or we just don't say anything at all and harbor resentment until it makes us sick in some way. Just as often, we hold back our natural creativity and unique spark for fear of what others will think. If we do not express the words that our hearts and minds generate, then we are not creating a life that is in accordance with our authentic selves.

There is a lack of coherence in not speaking the truth. When you hold back your truth—or when you tell an untruth—that is energy that has shifted out of your center and into some kind of off-lying vibration. That creates dissonant waveforms that are going to undermine the health of your thyroid and your system overall.

Thyroid medication is the number-one prescribed medication in the United States, which says volumes about the collective condition of our throat chakras—and how well programmed we have been by our culture to not be in truth. Women and minority groups in particular have been weakened and oppressed in this area. There's been a gagging and stunting of our natural expression that shows up in an inability to speak our truth as well as in the denial and suppression of our own emotions.

From what I have observed, the health of the thyroid is directly related to our communication habits. The thyroid, the gland connected with the throat chakra, is a little butterfly-shaped gland that sits right at the front of the base of the neck. Many thyroid-related disorders have to do with what we are saying or not saying. That might seem like an oversimplification, but in my experience, it's not. People with thyroid issues tend to have a profile of poor personal boundaries and a lack of self-advocacy and self-respect. They fail to speak their needs and desires, often bending over backward for everyone else at the detriment of themselves.

A majority of people have a somewhat unhealthy thyroid, whether they've been diagnosed or not. In my observation, most people have a significant amount of energy piling up on either side of their throats—meaning that the energy isn't flowing through the throat and energizing the thyroid. That pattern lays down the vibrational template for thyroid issues. When too much energy is stuck out on the right side of the throat—in speaking but not being heard—we can end up with hyperthyroidism. If we spend too much time on the left, stifling and not expressing ourselves, we end up with hypothyroidism, an underactive thyroid. If we express truth in the moment with kindness, love, respect, and diplomacy, we end up with healthy thyroidism.

You can take this or that medication for your thyroid, but it will not address the root of the problem. Your thyroid will heal the more you relax your body and become present in your truth, and the more your own voice vibrates your thyroid when you speak in a clear mid-tone range—which is the natural way we speak when we are relaxed and centered. Through that resonant vibration, the mechanical energy that comes from the center of your throat keeps the thyroid healthy.

Most thyroid issues are autoimmune, which speaks to the inner conflict of self against self. It's the self-censoring and self-judging self against the free, creative, emotional self. It takes a lot more energy to be two or more people inside of you than it does to be one. The divide-and-conquer that we see externalized in our culture is starting in an internalized place where most people have been inwardly divided against themselves. Instead of experiencing ourselves as a unified being that enjoys internal consensus, we are an inner critic divided against an inner victim. The thyroid speaks to that divide-and-conquer more than anything. I experienced this for years when I was bulimic: A part of me was saying, *Stop, stop, stop,* and another part was not able or not choosing to stop. The struggle of that lack of alignment between your behavior and your values is utterly exhausting, and it takes you out of the resonance of truth.

The key to thyroid health, as I see it, is speaking only truth and living in harmony with your truth. The truth is a good place to hang out! Living in truth with a functioning thyroid does wonders for our overall battery meter. We get more miles out of our tank of gas each day. I find that the more I'm flowing with the truth of who I am, the more I feel like a star flowing through the heavens. I'm just letting that truth guide my thoughts, words, and actions. Commit to speaking, writing, and expressing only truth. The more you do it, the better you get at it! Your thyroid will thank you.

I will be the first to acknowledge, however, that this isn't the easiest task. Most of us are afraid, to some extent, to speak our truth. Truth-tellers get punished. People who speak the truth tend to get ridiculed, and people who lie are often rewarded. It's been that way for millennia. This is a genuine and valid fear. We need to acknowledge our ancestors who were punished for speaking their truths, and we can start small in our own lives, finding places in which we're not centered in our truths and working to realign ourselves there. Ask yourself: What's a truth that you've been needing to confront with someone? What's a truth that you've been avoiding within yourself?

Here's a common example of a moment out of truth: A friend asks you to help them with something—moving, let's say—but you're tired, you don't have time, and you don't really want to. But you've been conditioned to be a people pleaser. You're supposed to be nice, so you say *yes* even when your body is saying *no.* The voice inside is a clear "I don't want to do that," but you don't know how to say *no* or you don't feel worthy of saying *no.* Or you're afraid of how they'll react. You override your body and say *yes.* It might seem like a small transgression, but when you tally all the little ways we dishonor our own needs, it adds up to big problems over time.

What if you don't know the voice of truth? When we have a lot of voices in our heads, it can be difficult to discern what's true. That's something you have to investigate for yourself over time. I've found that if I follow the guidance of my mail slot, things work out. And if I disregard something from the mail slot, afterward I often have a sense of *Shit, I should have done that.* Nobody else can tell you which is the right voice in your head. With some self-inquiry, you develop the discernment to know which voice leads to good outcomes and which voice leads to bad outcomes. Do those outcomes contribute to greater health, happiness, and harmony? Then that voice is leading you to your truth. Or do the outcomes you're creating lead to feeling ashamed, frustrated, or lacking? Then that voice is an ego-based construct that isn't beneficial. (And chances are it's the punitive voice of a parent that's still echoing in your head!)

For me, the truth feels like an upwelling. That's how I recognize it. It wells up inside me and wants to come out. In the first year that I was giving Biofield Tuning sessions, I would have all kinds of cues drop into my mind. Often they were very weird! I'd tell myself, *I'm not going to say that! That's so weird.* But it would keep coming back. Then it would get in the way of me being able to pay attention in the next moment. I discovered that I had to say these things! Otherwise, they'd bounce around in my head like a pinball, and eventually, I'd just have to spit them out. So I would say the weird thing to the person—and it would actually mean something to them. They'd get some benefit from receiving the message, and they'd be happy that I said it. I learned from that process to speak my truth in the moment as it arose. Now it's much easier for me to hear my guidance and discern what is my truth.

LEFT SIDE: THAT WHICH WE DO NOT SPEAK OR EXPRESS

When we habitually bite our tongues, hold back our emotions, stifle our natural expressions, and resist our own truths, energy builds up on the left side of the throat chakra. If you'd had a tendency in your life to not speak up for yourself and to not express your emotions or needs, energy pools and accumulates in this part of your field. There can be a sense of strangulation here—a feeling like it's not okay to express yourself. If you're someone who grew up in a home where children were to be seen but not heard, the result can be an energetic suppression of your ability to speak up. It can create a real knot in the flow of energy in the throat chakra.

The left side of the throat is a very suppressive place. Here we find the imprint of things that arise in us to be expressed, but were never spoken or otherwise released. Like the sacral area, this region is a big hub for repressed emotions to congregate and create drag on the system. I often encounter energy here that moves like molasses in January. It's just incredibly thick, heavy, and slow-moving. Energy accumulates out here when we bite our tongues; when we hold back our feelings, desires, needs, or even our ideas and visions. It could be something as simple as holding back a swear when you stub your toe. When an impulse to express is generated in the body, that is a thing that has an actual mass. If it doesn't come out, it has to go somewhere—and it ends up out there in your field, sequestering your life force.

It takes a lot of energy to hold our emotions back—much more than the amount of energy required to let things out. When we suppress expression from the throat chakra, we deny passage of that emotion through this energy center, which means that the thyroid isn't getting the juice it needs to run properly. This really lowers our voltage. In fact, I think it's one of the most destructive things that we can do for our health. Why? Because what doesn't come out stays in. Until we release that energy, it's going to stick around and cause problems. Those impulses lodge in our field, creating static and distortion.

A pattern of stunted emotional expression often goes back to early childhood. Everyone's parents had a phrase that they used to stop them from being emotional—for my parents, it was, "Stop your nonsense!" We're not allowed to express our emotions, so we learn to internalize our expression. We start to feel guilty for feeling, and we come to fear our own emotions. The child who made the decision not to feel something remains the reference point in adulthood. But once the emotion is given room to play itself out, it's never as bad as we think it's going to be. It's never as scary or horrible as our fear tells us it is. I see people suppress emotions because the emotion feels so big that they're afraid it will never end. But in my years of working on the emotional body—my own and that of others—I have yet to encounter an infinite, bottomless emotion. They all have ends and bottoms.

When people have a strong habit of self-censoring, energy can pile up very densely around four inches off the side of the throat. Here we find a structure in the biofield anatomy known as the *throat filter*. This structure acts like a filter for energy, catching the things we don't say and hanging on to them. It reminds me of the lint trap in my dryer. When I was teaching in England, I was astonished by the amount of lint I was finding in people's throat filters. It was nearly twice as thick as what I'd seen in Americans. Health is flow, and we want to get our *words* into a flow state so that we can start living our lives in a flow state. Every time you let your words flow instead of stopping yourself short, you energetically clean out your throat filter. Let whatever wants to come out, come out—just do it in a way that's kind and respectful. I've treated a number of people with vertigo and Ménière's disease successfully by helping them to clean up this area. It seems like when it is really overloaded it can actually make us dizzy!

This is really an act of reclaiming our wildness. We are wild creatures! Have you ever been around kids? What do they like to do? They like to run around and dance and make noise. But what we're forced to do in school is sit down and shut up. This puts a big hurting on our throat chakras. It's like we've all got dirty sweat socks stuck in our mouths. We're not free in the throat, and so much of it is our conditioning from school. Many of us got a lot of punishment around our voices in school. Not only do we have this fear of being yelled at, we're afraid of being wrong. *I'm going to say the wrong thing. I'm going to be humiliated. I'm going to speak out of turn. I'm going to get punished.*

I see in so many people a desire to howl at the moon, to roar, to vocalize our wildness that's been swallowed and internalized and often turned into depression. It's a very damp, muted energy. The feeling I often get in my own body when feeling into these areas is very restricted, almost like I'm wearing a straitjacket. Don't mistake the programming of domesticity for the truth of who you are. Reclaim that inner roar. The roar is a metaphor for life, creation, expression, your truth. In Buddhism, the lion's roar is a metaphor for the power of speaking the spiritual truths of the dharma. For all of us, it's a potent symbol of the power of expressing our truths.

In 2017, I had the good fortune of meeting the legendary jazz musician Herbie Hancock. Herbie told me that before each show, he and his band gather backstage and take a moment to chant with intention—and their intention is for their audience to have the *courage to express themselves!* This is a wonderful intention to experiment with for yourself and to send out into the collective.

RIGHT SIDE: SPEAKING BUT NOT BEING HEARD

The right side of the throat records information related to when we're speaking but not being heard. If you were left to cry it out as an infant, or if you had a neglectful or absent parent, there's a lot of information that will get encoded in this area very early on. If you weren't listened to or if your needs weren't being met when you were very young, you will likely form beliefs like: *Nobody cares what I have to say. It doesn't matter what I think. It doesn't matter what I want. Everyone else's needs matter, and mine don't.*

It's really hard to not be heard! I've worked with many people who are trying their darndest to communicate whatever their version of truth is, but it's just not being received by the people in their lives. Having a spouse, a mother or father, or a boss who doesn't listen to you is a tough thing to deal with. An ongoing pattern of being ignored or misunderstood by lots of people in your life is even tougher. This kind of patterning creates a lot of tension to the right of the throat, often paired with a frustration over unmet needs spinning down in the left hip.

This is also something we're really struggling with as a culture right now. We're all yelling at each other, and nobody's listening! In our politics and public discourse, there's so much division and so many people falling on one side of an issue or the other, and a lot of hunkering down and not listening and being angry about not being heard. The good news is that when we work on this patterning in ourselves, we're also helping to work on it in the collective. If people were listening better and being heard more, things would be working a lot better.

Imbalances in the right side of the throat aren't just about our ability to communicate with others. There's an area around four inches off the right side of the throat where energy piles up when we speak to *ourselves* but don't listen. Your body, your higher self or your conscience—the part of you that knows what you need to be doing to be healthy, emotionally, physically, spiritually—is speaking to you all the time. Can you hear it underneath the noise of your monkey mind? Are you responding to that guidance or are you ignoring it?

I think we all have an internal cue dropper that guides us to "say this" or "don't do that." I used to always wonder how jazz musicians get together and jam, coordinate themselves so effortlessly to create a dynamic piece of music on the spot. How do they know what to play next? If you talk to a jazz musician, they will tell you that it's because the note drops in a half-beat ahead of time. The cue drops in, and the player follows without question or hesitation. It's the same with our own inner cues. The part of us that is directing our little avatar here and is saying, "Go here. Do that. Say this. Finish this first." That cue dropper is the voice of your inner authority—your conscience, your higher self, whatever you want to call it. Maybe even God or Source. Either we listen to those subtle cues and we do what they ask of us, or we ignore them. Over time, disregarding the cues comes at a cost. When we listen to the cues, we're in greater harmony with other players in the game of life. When we disregard those cues, we get out of sync with ourselves, with others and with all of life.

If you want to be heard by others, the best thing you can do is learn to listen to yourself. The more you listen to and respond to your own inner authority, the more *outer* authority you're going to have with other people. If you want to make a difference in the world, you need to be in integrity with your own inner guidance. The more you listen to yourself and honor and respect yourself, the more other people will listen to you, honor you, and respect you. When you're being heard and respected, it's much easier to extend that same courtesy to other people. You will become more powerful and influential because you have credibility with yourself. A good mantra to use here is simply, *I'm heard*. Or if that's too much, you can say, *I like it when I'm heard. It feels good to be heard*—that one is certainly true! You can also say, *I listen to and honor myself*, and *I'm worthy of whatever cues are dropping in right now*.

Another huge factor in determining how people respond to you is your tone of voice. Tones carry information about our emotions and subconscious beliefs. When you're speaking your truth from a place of inner authority, that information is reflected in your tone of voice. When you carry a belief like, *It doesn't matter what I say, nobody is listening and nobody cares*, that information is also reflected in the tone of your voice—and other people will respond accordingly. It's been said that in communication, 10 percent of what determines how people respond to you is your words, 20 percent is your body language, and 70 percent is your tone of voice. The tone is the *feeling*, the resonance, behind the words. You recognize the sadness of a song not just from the lyrics but from the tone of the notes being played.

I am always amazed how much a person's tone of voice can change after some adjustments are done on their throat chakra. I've worked with many singers and speakers who tell me that the tonality of their voices improve, sometimes dramatically, when they do this work. As they release tension in the thyroid and vagus nerve, as their whole systems relax into a more coherent expression, their voices becomes more resonant as a consequence. And as we all know, it's much more pleasing to listen to a voice that's resonant and balanced rather than one that's tight or faint.

Where does that tone come from? The larynx, which is the main biological apparatus that you use to create sound, is animated by the vagus nerve, which connects the heart, lungs, and digestive tract to the brain. If you have tension in your liver, your tone of voice is going to come through with that angry edge. If your kidneys are all bunched up, you'll have that breathless fear in your voice. Whatever is going on as far as patterns of tension goes, it's going to show up in the tone of your voice. When you're relaxed, your voice is more resonant because there are more open resonant cavities in your body. When there's tension, it makes things all thin and high. Paying attention to tone of voice is a great way to tell how much tension a person is holding, what their underlying emotional baseline is, and what beliefs they carry. Notice how when you're being ignored, that creates tension in the body. That tension becomes a pattern as it continually gets retriggered over time.

The other side of the equation is listening to other people more deeply and carefully. When we extend the courtesy of deep listening, it's much more likely to be reciprocated. We can't just go into automatic invalidation. Instead of me trying to invalidate my husband's perspective on something to validate my own, I can look at the issue from his perspective and say, "Oh, yeah, you're right. From your perspective, it really does look different." Letting them be right doesn't make you wrong. Again, it's a *both-and* rather than *either-or*.

There's a quote I love from Johan Boswinkel, a brilliant Dutch scientist who invented a biophoton device for healing. He says, "Truth has 144 sides." When I first heard this, it stuck in my head like an arrow, and I puzzled over its meaning for days. The more I thought about it, the more I've realized that we can only ever see one perspective on things, and it's really important to realize that "the truth, the whole truth, and nothing but the truth" for me is going to be different from what it is for you. It's important that we be willing to listen to another person's perspective and honor that and realize that the truth is prismatic, and we are just reflecting different sides of truth.

SUCCESSFUL DIPLOMACY

When you're living in the transparency of truth, you're free to say what needs to be said in the moment—and here's the kicker—to do it *without putting out a charge*. If you put out charge, you're going to get back charge. We need to learn to let out these things that arise, but in a way that we can feel good about. There's a diplomacy to be learned in all of this.

When we're able to handle frustrations and discomforts on the spot, we stop them from turning big and ugly. "Confrontation" isn't necessary when we speak without charge, when we come from a position of respect and kindness. This is what I call *successful diplomacy*. There's a good chance you never learned it from your parents, as most of us grew up with models of communication that were either scary or ineffectual, so we need to figure out for ourselves what it means to express our needs, opinions, and desires in a way that is firm but kind.

Successful diplomacy is something you can teach yourself. The way to do that is generally through trial and error—and I won't lie, the error part hurts. Speaking from experience, it can *really* sting. You try to speak your truth, and it comes out in the wrong way. I've seen many people decide that they won't speak their truth because they tried, and well, look at the carnage that was created! But you have to be committed to it. Do a note to self for next time when you communicate in a way that's not effective, and then let it go.

You have to be willing to go through a messy period as you learn successful diplomacy, but it's a skill that is worthwhile to learn. Holding on to hurt, to unsaid words, keeps us stuck in the past and unable to be fully present for this moment and creates a big drag on our overall electric health. If this is new territory for you, a good place to start is the book *Nonviolent Communication: A Language of Compassion* by Marshall B. Rosenberg. Another system we have made use of in my organization is *Crucial Conversations* (available as both a book and an online training program), which outlines how to approach difficult situations with diplomacy and effectiveness.

YOUR POWER AS A CREATOR

The ultimate expression of the throat is not just to communicate effectively but to step into our true power as the authors and creators of our own lives.

The word is creative! We hear this over and over, but it doesn't sink in. Everything you say is an affirmation. Everything you think is an affirmation. When you say things like, *I'm broke,* and *I'm sick,* or any kind of *I am* statement, you are creating that. You might create it immediately, or you might create it over time. But when you're disconnected from the words that you are thinking and speaking, and what you're saying isn't reflecting the truth of who you are, then you're not creating a life that has anything to do with who you really are.

It's so important to be mindful of the stories you're telling yourself about who you are and what you can and can't do. Those stories are just programming that can be reprogrammed. You are the storyteller, and you can change the story whenever you decide to. If you want to get the junk out of your life, stop speaking junk. If you want to be prosperous, if you want to be abundant, if you want to be healthy and strong, you have to speak and think all those things. I have learned to never sit around going, "I'm so fat, I'm so broke, I'm struggling." I've done that. When I was saying those words, that was my reality.

Sometimes we can have blind spots around this and habitual subconscious ways of creating without realizing it. As silly as it sounds, I did this with my hair. After losing a bunch of hair from a CT scan in 2012, it was never the same, and it became brittle and frizzy and annoying. I kept on saying, "I hate my hair," until my son Cassidy pointed out to me what I was doing and the power of my word. So I decided to start saying, "I love my hair" (even though I really didn't), and I kept saying it. In a short time, I finally found both a good hairdresser who knew what to do with my hair and a product that actually got rid of the frizz. And suddenly, I really did love my hair! There *will* be lag time between your words and what shows up, and a lot of people give up before things shift. Don't give up!

There's a great little book by Charles Capp called *The Tongue: A Creative Force*. In it, there's a quote, attributed to Christ, that says, "I have told my people they can have what they say. But my people keep saying what they have." I always say that if you go to a restaurant and you don't ask for what you want, you're going to get bread and water. A lot of people's lives are bread and water. If we could more clearly articulate our intentions and desires, if we could ask for what we really wanted, it could be delivered to us.

The best way to become more powerful as a creator is to keep your word. Every time you say you're going to do something and then you don't do it, your energy dissipates. You lose power. The energy of your throat weakens. When you're not in integrity with your word and your deed—when there's a gap between what you say you're going to do and what you actually do—you diminish your ability to create. A little magic tip: If you want to be powerful, you have to do what you say you're going to do. Because every time you do what you say you're going to, you instill your word with integrity and power. You believe yourself. You know that if you say you're going to do something, you'll do it. That gives you an authority with yourself that others then respond to, which increases your ability to manifest through what you're thinking and speaking. A couple of good affirmations here are *I keep my word* and *I don't speak my word until I'm ready to keep it.*

THE CREATIVE WORD: PROSPERITY AND ABUNDANCE

Your relationship with money is a great place to start playing around with the creative power of your word. I have found that abundance has a great deal to do with what we speak about money. Many people stay in the same financial situation for their whole lives, and that has everything to do with the stories they're telling themselves.

Our (often subconscious) beliefs about money are almost like religious beliefs. We get *really* stuck in them. They form very tight patterns in our fields. As children, we didn't have beliefs about money. Our parents imparted to us our first beliefs about what money is and the role it plays in our lives. They create in us a distorted lens through which we perceive something, money, that's essentially neutral—just a form of energy, a currency, like anything else.

What stories are getting in the way of you living an abundant life? Do you have a story that you can't trust yourself or the universe? Do you have a story of not being taken care of? Or a story of separation, isolation, and lack? Those stories can and often do block cash flow. But it's all just static, and when that static goes away, we recognize the clear truth that we simply *are* abundant as part of nature and a part of the human race.

You are abundant in cells! You're abundant in microorganisms. You're abundant in plasma.

Here are a few common money stories that don't do us a whole lot of good: *Money is the root of all evil. Money is dirty. Money doesn't matter to me. Caring about money is materialistic. If I have more money, other people have less. The money we need won't be there when I need it. It's nobler to give money than it is to receive it.* These are mind viruses, plain and simple! They're beliefs. They're stories. Money is just energy! It's neutral in itself. How we feel about money is often a reflection of how we feel about life itself.

Changing the story changes the feeling, the resonance, and the emotional tone we carry around money, which attracts different experiences and outcomes. The emotion attached to what you're saying is even more important than the words themselves. When you say, "I'm broke," you're evoking that feeling of being broke, and then that feeling is what's being attracted to those experiences in your life. An emotion creates a magnetic field that attracts like energies into your field. When I say that I'm abundant, there's a feeling that's attached to that: a feeling of connectivity, expansiveness, and fullness. I'm connected to the universe, and the universe is abundant. Ultimately, the number of digits that appear in your online statement have nothing to do with whether you are attuned to and aligned with the essential abundant nature of being.

You may have to fake it till you make it. There's nothing wrong with that! You have to be willing to experiment with feeling abundant even if your bank account may be telling you something different. See if you can find a way to feel abundant without any regard to your cash flow situation. Are you abundant in love? In gratitude? In nonfinancial sources of support? You'll find that the more you feel abundant, the more people smile at you. Interesting things come your way that aren't necessarily a check in the mail. Somebody just gave you a gift out of nowhere or someone did you a favor.

Here is a little story of manifestation and abundance that just happened to me: One of the things I have been experimenting with here in Jamaica is using straight aloe leaf on my skin as a moisturizer every day (it's been working amazingly well!). A couple of days ago, I decided that I also wanted to experiment with smearing pineapple on my face and see what that did. So yesterday when I went to town, I was planning on getting a pineapple. However, I forgot, because I was so engrossed in writing at the beach that I didn't notice the time, and I had to hurry back for my appointment with my massage therapist, who conveniently lives right behind me.

As I was emerging from the massage and walking up the driveway to where her mother has a little shop, there was a station wagon full of all kinds of fresh produce, and folks were buying things from it. One of my Jamaican friends was standing there, and as I walked past the car, he said, "Do you want a pineapple?" I said, "Yes, I do actually, but I don't have any cash." And he said, "No worries. I will buy the pineapple for you."

He didn't ask me about bananas or papayas or mangoes. For whatever reason, he seemed quite determined to buy me a pineapple. So I let him, and I came home with the gifted pineapple. These are the kinds of things that happen to us as we start to feel more abundant and magnetic!

A good way to practice shifting your feelings around money is to tune in to your self-talk and especially *how you feel* when you're paying your bills. Pay attention to that feeling of going to write a big check that you don't want to write. Notice what your thoughts are as you get that constricted, uncomfortable feeling. Everything is sucking in toward you because you're feeling fear and lack and scarcity. This is where we flip the script. What if you said to yourself, *I'm so fortunate that I have the money to be able to pay this bill. I'm lucky that I'm able to pay my rent.* When you write a check for those car repairs, you feel relaxed and grateful, you feel a flow-through of your energy instead of feeling all tense and bunched up. That's a very different approach! One of the single best things you can do around money is to learn to let go of it with a sense of ease and gratitude and flow. Be grateful that you have the money to spend. When we change the dialogue, I've found that the feeling is generally pretty quick to follow.

Working with your own beliefs around money isn't just about you getting to a place where you can take fancier vacations and buy a nicer car (though I don't object to those things). This is also about the greater good. When we tell ourselves stories about money being bad, we rob ourselves of the potential of maximizing the good we can do in the world. The more money we have, the more good things we can do. What happens when kind, conscious people don't make money their friend is that we end up with a lot of good-hearted people with little power to enact change in the world. Imagine if people with compassion and integrity also had the ability to move some serious capital around! How different would the world be? People would get fed. Communities would be supported. Our lives would be enriched by the arts. Let's liberate money from where it's stuck and get it into the hands of artists and musicians and healers and storytellers and small farmers.

You don't have to reject money. You can love money, knowing that it helps you to be a force for good in the world. Speak kindly to money. Invite it into your life. Magnetize money to yourself so that you can spread it around in a happy way. Tell it, "Hey, money, I think you're cool. I'd love to hang out and see what we can do together." There's much more that I could say about this, but for now, I refer you again to Ken Honda's book *Happy Money*, which does an excellent job of describing how to make money your friend.

Plant seeds with your words, fertilize those seeds with your intention and attention, and watch as they grow into the garden of a life that is in tune with the truth of your being.

15

THIRD EYE:
Widening the Lens

The third eye, or brow, energy center—located between the eyebrows and governing the brain, physical eyes, and pineal gland—relates to our intuition and thought processes. When balanced, it brings mental clarity, focus, insight, trust, and surrender, as well as an ability to see the bigger picture of life. A clear flow of energy through this center leads to greater presence in the moment, peace of mind, connection to one's intuition, inner guidance, and visionary capacity, as well as a greater awareness of our own gifts and purpose in life. The third eye resonates on the spectrum of visible light as the color indigo, and as a sound wave, it is the note A and the sound "AUM" or "OM" (in Vedic cosmology, the primordial sound that brought the whole universe into being).

The third eye is often romanticized for its connection to the mystical and psychic realms, but from my perspective, it has more to do with our *ability to be in the present moment*. When the mind is centered in the now, we are able to see this moment clearly for what it is—instead of seeing through the distorted lens of our old beliefs, stories, and judgments. *Clairvoyance* (translation: "clear seeing") is the natural result of showing up for the moment with a beginner's mind. It's delightfully simple. It is when we are fully in the moment, deeply attuned to our inner and outer environments, that we receive visions, intuitive hits, and subtle magnetic guidance. When the third eye is fully open and on line, we're seeing exactly what we need to see, when we need to see it. We have the clarity to look beyond our own illusions to the truth of the moment.

I find that imbalances in the third eye are caused by things like overthinking, worrying about the future, regretting the past, not being able to discern truth, doubting our own perception and inclinations, memory problems, concussions, and PTSD. When the third eye is blocked, we can experience mental fuzziness, brain fog, an inability to focus, uncertainty and doubt, and a sense of disconnection from our own inner guidance systems.

Post-traumatic stress often results in extreme imbalances in the third eye. In people who suffer from PTSD, I frequently encounter a cloud of thick energy and audible static from the edge of the field all the way to the head on both the right and left sides. It feels to me like being in a large house with all the lights and appliances turned on in every room. There's so much neural activity that the person can barely handle any more input because there's no brainpower left to process it. I've found sound work to be highly effective in turning down the noise in the brain and allowing it to return to normal functioning.

Not only post-traumatic stress but any mental habits and thought patterns that take us *out* of the moment block the clear signal of the third eye. A mind that is not in the present moment is a mind in the past or the future. The left side of the third eye is where I find patterns of worry and anticipation about the future. There's a structure roughly ten inches off the left side of the head that I call the *hamster wheel of worry*, which gets energized when the mind starts running off into concerns over how we're going to pay the bills, whether our businesses are going to survive, what to do about so-and-so, whether that headache is actually a brain tumor, and so on. The right side is where energy spins when we're dwelling on the past. Around ten inches off the right side of the forehead, we hit the *hamster wheel of regret*, which is driven by thoughts of remorse, guilt, and shame: *If only, I should have, I shouldn't have, I was better back then.* This reflection is typically negative but sometimes can reflect an excessive preoccupation with the "good old days."

We all have within us the capacity to be a visionary: to be given dreams, visions, and missions and to have enough clarity to know the next steps and to get the cues to execute them. But we've got to be in the now if we want to do that. The effect of running these hamster wheels and getting ourselves all twisted up and torquing between our right and left brain hemispheres is that we're not centered in the present. When we're indulging a preoccupation with the past and future, we're not in the clear vibration of the now.

In the biofield anatomy, the back of the third eye center holds information about our physical eyes as well as the imprint of things sitting around in the metaphorical "back of your head." It's also about opening up and *receiving* clairvoyance, creative inspiration, sudden downloads. What are you letting in to your awareness? What new ideas, visions, and inspirations are entering into you and inspiring you? The mantra here is "I'm open." *I'm open to receiving whatever information I need to receive in this moment. I'm open to seeing with new eyes. I'm open to seeing new solutions to old problems.*

With the ability to change our perception, we have the power to change our reality. I've worked with thousands of people and witnessed many personal transformations—and there isn't one that didn't start with a shift of perspective. Often it starts small. I recall one particular Biofield Tuning session in which I discovered some very heavy static in my client's third eye. We spent over an hour clearing it with the forks. She emailed me the next day to say that when she woke up in the morning, she looked around her home and said to herself, *What's all this junk? What are all these boxes and stacks of magazines? That's not supposed to be here.* Once her mind was clear, she found a new clarity on how the clutter in her environment had been creating noise in her mind and vice versa. The shift in perspective led to a new behavior, which created a tangible change in her life.

YOUR MAGNETIC SENSE

The cool thing is that when we wire our brains to operate in the present moment, we also cultivate our innate capacity for extrasensory perception.

The gland associated with the third eye is the pineal gland, named such for its resemblance to a pine cone. Located right in the center of your forehead, your pineal gland, like your two eyes, has rods and cones for receiving light. It's no wonder that so many cultures throughout history have referred to it as the "inner eye." It is, in fact, a kind of visual apparatus! I often experience it as a little purple light bulb radiating out from the middle of the brain. My sense is that the light frequencies perceived by the pineal gland are from higher wavelengths of energy that pass through the skull, only to be seen through the mind's eye. Think of it as *perceiving* all the light we cannot see. When the pineal gland is awake and fully on line, we are highly attuned to the finer frequencies that surround us. We are able to receive and interpret the information carried on those frequencies and to use that information to guide us through the world.

The pineal gland governs what I've come to think of as our magnetic sense. It's like an antenna that's constantly picking up subtle electromagnetic signaling, and as such, it is connected to our ability to perceive cosmic and earthly vibrational information. It's often said that the pineal gland is our connection to God or spirit. I describe it as our connection to the universe—the universe being this electromagnetic organism of which we are each one tiny individual cell. Like any of the cells in our own bodies, we want there to be a sense of unification with the one central organizing intelligence that everything in our bodies are attuned to.

An attuned pineal gland is attentive to the music of the spheres and our own consequent steps in the cosmic dance. When the pineal gland is activated, when we're fully in the now, we're open to the magnetic vibes of the universe and we're in tune with the Schumann resonance, the electromagnetic pulse of the earth. This constant background pulse that is occurring within the earth's iconic cavity seems to act as a metronome for the pineal gland, which then becomes the basis for all our circadian rhythms.

Both ancient spiritual belief and contemporary neuroscience have associated pineal gland activity with intuition, clairvoyance, and so-called psychic, or extrasensory, abilities. Extrasensory perception isn't so mysterious when it comes right down to it. It's just the natural and healthy expression of the pineal gland. The research of UC–Berkeley-trained biophysicist Beverly Rubik found that the brain region located right around the pineal gland consistently operates at 40 Hz, a high frequency associated with intuition and clairvoyance as well as love, gratitude, and child-like wonder. These qualities are our natural state as children. We saw things, and we knew things. We talked to ghosts and invisible friends. We exhibited what might be called *psychic behavior.* If the adults in your life freaked out or scolded you when you shared those perceptions, there's a good chance you shut those abilities down. Even if they didn't, you likely began to invalidate and shut them down on your own as you got older and realized that they didn't fit into the materialist worldview you were being taught.

When my boys were around five and eight years old, I discovered that they could see people's energy fields. They saw colors around almost everyone, and they were very surprised that I couldn't see them too. Years later, in their early teens, I remember asking them if they still saw colors around people, and they said, "Nah, not really." Somewhere along the way, that perception was lost—and it certainly wasn't because their mother told them it was weird! There are so many reasons that we shut down these innate gifts. But they can be turned back on. A big first step is the knowledge that these extra-perceptual abilities being in the on position is their balanced, harmonious expression.

These abilities are also connected to what scientists call *magneto-reception:* the sensory ability of an organism to detect magnetic fields in order to perceive direction, altitude, or location. Sea turtles, migrating birds, eels, dolphins, foxes, bees, and even certain strains of bacteria (potentially *all* organisms, in fact) use the earth's magnetic fields for navigation. It's the homing device sea turtles use to navigate across vast expanses of open ocean and return to the same beach where they hatched, to lay their own eggs. It's how flocks of hundreds of starlings come together in a breathtaking synchronized dance across the sky. Monarch butterflies use their magnetic compasses to stay on course during cloudy and overcast days when migrating south to Mexico. Magnetotactic bacteria migrate along the field lines of the earth's magnetic field using magnetite, a chemical that's been found in the pineal gland and throughout the human brain.

All of nature has a magnetic sense. I just read an article, in fact, about how dogs poop in alignment with the earth's magnetic field! It's just part of life. We humans are not any different from the rest of nature. By one recent estimate, the pineal gland is made up of 30 percent magnetite, a naturally occurring mineral that is sensitive to magnetic fields. But it's not just the physical brain that's picking up magnetic information. We even have magnetoreceptors in our eyes—we can literally see magnetic fields! This magnetic sense was well utilized by preindustrial humans. Native peoples around the world had the ability to navigate unimaginable distances without a map or compass—often in the total absence of visual cues in the landscape.

It wasn't until the 1990s that scientists discovered for the first time that the brain contains these magnetic particles. The researchers quickly ruled out the possibility that the particles were caused by magnetic pollution—the fact that every brain studied had a similar distribution of the magnetic particles suggested that they served a biological function. Because the particles were more concentrated in lower regions of the brain and tapered off in higher regions, the researchers hypothesized that they likely played a role in helping electrical signals travel from the spine up and into the brain.

Still, the scientific consensus was that humans did not have a magnetic sense. That stance was dealt a major blow in 2019, when a group of researchers at the California Institute of Technology found, for the first time, conclusive neuroscientific proof of a human geomagnetic navigation system. When the researchers shifted the magnetic field of a testing chamber, EEG measurements of the study participants' brain activity revealed that certain magnetic rotations triggered strong and reproducible brain responses. Alpha brain wave amplitude dropped suddenly—a response that typically occurs when a person suddenly detects a new sensory stimuli. All of this was operating on a subconscious level, however, and the participants were unaware of the magnetic shifts and the changes in their own brain activity. As the study's authors explained: "We've found evidence that people have working magnetic sensors sending signals to the brain—a previously unknown sensory ability in the subconscious human mind. The full extent of our magnetic inheritance remains to be discovered."

This "magnetic inheritance" is an innate ability that anyone can develop and cultivate. The ability to be attuned to our ambient magnetic environment, to feel where the flow of life is taking us, is an ability that has been lost in many modern humans—and yet is key to being in a state of flow and thereby health. We were born with an inner GPS. We have within our bodies an electromagnetic compass that is aligned with the magnetic field of the earth and is pointing at all times in the direction of our own true north. This natural potential isn't gone, we've just become disconnected from it. We've been told that we can only perceive what we see, so we haven't thought to look further. We've had blinders on against it. But once you know that you have this perceptual ability that's as natural to you as your senses of sight and smell, you can start to tap into it. If you know it and trust it, then you will experience it. If you don't know it's possible and you don't believe it, then you won't even look for it.

There's a simple meditation I like to use to connect with my magnetic sense. Take a moment to center yourself, and see if you can sense into a bright purple light between your eyebrows. Feel it radiating out from the center of your head in all directions like a lighthouse. Then slowly start to expand your awareness from the center of your head to the space around you. Slowly widen your awareness to encompass the magnetic bubble that surrounds you. Feel yourself inside that bubble. Feel that bubble inside the earth's bubble, which is also inside the sun's bubble. Feel into the sun's bubble inside the galaxy's magnetic bubble. Feel your connection to all the resonance of waves traveling within all these bubbles: your own body, the earth, the sun, the galaxy. Allow your awareness to expand, merging with the awareness of the universe. Allow your antenna, your pineal gland, to be exquisitely attuned to this field of vibrational reality of infinite frequencies. Feel that antenna opening up to cosmic waves from the center of the universe, from the sun and stars, from Source itself. Hear and feel the pulse of the Schumann resonance. Allow it to guide you in the direction you need to go in your life. If you use your voice as an instrument, this is a great space to practice resonating the different frequencies using your imagination.

STAYING HEALTHY IN AN ELECTROMAGNETIC ENVIRONMENT

When the pineal gland isn't functioning properly, it's often because it's become overcharged as a result of picking up too much electromagnetic information. Electromagnetic static in our environment acts as signal jammers for our own antennas to receive true, subtler signals from nature.

When I'm working on this energy center, I often find clusters of noise and debris that I liken to space junk—those metal pieces of old satellites floating around the earth's atmosphere. It's a heavy load of interference. This often creates a stressful sense of impaired perception and disconnection from one's environment—not unlike the experience of having one of our other senses impaired. I recently spent a few days with a friend of mine who has 50 percent hearing loss and wears a hearing aid, and I noticed how stressful it was for her to not be able to hear what was going on and to miss what people were saying. When our magnetic sense is blocked, too, there's a straining of our consciousness as we struggle to attune to the energy around us. We want to address this signal jamming, because it prevents us from tuning in to more harmonious and beneficial vibrations. Once we remove this noise, a sense of clarity and relaxation returns.

Enhancing our electrical health means improving the signal-to-noise ratio of all the body's electronics. The stronger our own signaling is, the higher the voltage in our bodies, the clearer our signals, the less we are impacted by all the noise in the environment. This is key to surviving in our present environment, where information is flowing all around us and through us in an ever-increasing electro-smog of conflicting signals.

Try bringing your awareness inside your head and see if you can feel or notice anything that might be going on and creating interference. Food allergies, heavy metal toxicity, and EMF sensitivity are all common issues here. If you're dealing with brain fog, poor memory, or an inability to focus, I encourage you to do some of your own research on these things and see if you can get a pulse on what might be going on for you. And of course, know that overthinking is often the biggest signal jammer of all!

LEFT SIDE: THE HAMSTER WHEEL OF WORRY

The imbalances I detect in the third eye are most frequently on the left side of the head, in the left brain hemisphere, which controls the right (yang) side of the body. Here we find patterns of future thinking, which often takes the form of compulsive worry, anxious spiraling, and negative anticipation. Sometimes it's the voice of an out-of-control inner taskmaster that's constantly repeating and rehashing your to-do list. Other times, it's a mental habit of escaping into an imagined future when we think we'll finally be happy. We talked about this kind of point-on-the-horizon, greener-pastures thinking in the knees chapter, and it's a huge pattern that also shows up in this part of the field. When we're caught up in this kind of thinking, we're not centered, grounded, or balanced energetically.

Roughly ten inches off the left side of the head, we find the energetic structure that I call the *hamster wheel of worry*. It's the male (yang) hamster spinning frantically on his little wheel, always running forward into the future. What's driving the hamster is the voice of *I gotta do this. I gotta do that. I gotta pay my taxes. I gotta send my kids to college. I gotta figure out my business. I gotta, I gotta, I gotta.* When this is going, we get frothy and project our energies out in front of us, into the future. We are outside the now when we're spinning that kind of energy. This hamster is connected with and fueling the wheel of guilt-driven overdoing at the right hip. Overthinking drives overdoing. Together, these two wheels are the primary source of energy leakage that I see in most people.

Sometimes it's not even just one hamster. Some people have multiple hamsters. I worked on a woman who had three, one of which was cock-eyed and running sideways! She had multiple voices going in her head all the time, and as a result, she suffered from terrible insomnia. We were able to slow down the hamsters by bringing awareness to those thought patterns and using the forks to reintegrate that stuck energy into the central channel, bringing her energy back into the now. Another time, I worked with a man who was having kidney trouble. It was apparent that the energy of his kidneys was very weak. What I discovered when I got into his field was that he had an unbelievably hyperactive hamster wheel on the left side of his head. In fact, I had never experienced such a zippy hamster! He was an overthinker, and his overthinking was pulling energy out of his kidneys and his entire body. The overthinking was driven by an old belief that he needed to figure everything out to protect himself and to be safe—a belief many people harbor that is simply not true.

When I was bulimic as a teenager, I drove myself crazy with the kind of forward-thinking energy that characterizes addictions of all kinds. I was constantly thinking about what I was going to eat, when I was going to eat it, and whether or not I was going to throw it up. We can have this kind of compulsive thinking about almost anything. Again tied to the wheel at the right hip, many people have it around work and productivity.

When we start thinking too much about the future, we spin out. It's not comfortable. It creates anxiety and tension, and we stop breathing. If you can just stay in the present moment with your breath, if you can just be in *this* moment, then you're okay. The way to get safely off the hamster wheel of racing thoughts is to become aware of what's happening so that you can catch yourself and return to the present. I'm not saying anything new here: This is mindfulness 101. When you become aware that your hamsters are running, that is a moment to breathe, center, and ground. Put your awareness in the middle of your forehead and center yourself back in the moment. Drop into your solar plexus or your heart if that feels right. Bring things back to now, and be grateful for what you have in this moment.

The other antidote to imbalances of future thinking is to learn to trust in your future self. If you don't trust your future self to manage the future, then you're going to feel the need to spend the present moment worrying about it. People who don't trust themselves often don't trust life. Or they don't trust what they've done in the past, and they believe that they always make mistakes. These are just stories that we need to interrogate. What if you could trust your future self to manage the moments that your future self is in? You don't need your past self to be managing everything and getting all bunched up trying to run the show before it's even begun. That doesn't mean that we don't plan. You might take your time every day to sit down and plan today or tomorrow or next week or next year to the extent that's appropriate for the situation. But once you've spent your time planning, scheduling, and writing things down, you don't need the hamster wheel running anymore.

RIGHT SIDE: RUNNING BACKWARD

The field to the right of the third eye—which correlates with the right brain hemisphere that controls the left side of the body—carries the more yin, feminine mental imbalance correlated with a more reflective, ruminative, backward-looking kind of thinking. This includes the inner critic, who is often giving us a hard time for something we did wrong in the past.

Much of the static here relates to things that we're having a hard time letting go of—the old grievances and old stories that are still running on repeat. Here, I often find charged-up memories that the mind is still looping in, as well as patches of trauma, difficulty, and intense inputs that are still acting as interrupters to our third eye perception. If there's an event from a person's life that they keep going back to again and again in their mind, the energy here will be very charged. The hamster wheel of regret is driven by a hamster who's running backward, looking to the past. An overactive female hamster—in other words, a tendency to dwell on the past—drives feelings of powerlessness, frustration, and victimhood that create charge and congestion around the left hip.

Running these hamsters is not sanity. It's not necessary, and it's not helpful. It creates a tremendous amount of signal jamming that clouds clear seeing, clear perception, and clear awareness. If your hamsters are out of control, that's a problem. They're *your* hamsters! If you're not in control of them, who is? You alone are responsible for whether these hamsters are behaving or not. It's up to you to own that. You have to exercise the discipline to notice when your hamsters are going rogue and to pull yourself back into the now.

OVERCOMING OVERTHINKING

We have to recognize that we've been programmed for overthinking. The reality is that most people go through life with a thinking mind that's driving them crazy. It hasn't always been that way—it's only in the past two hundred years or so that this unhealthy "thinking mind" construct has become a part of our reality. Over generations, we've seen the seat of consciousness shift from the solar plexus and the heart up into the head and the brain—which is not where most traditional cultures saw or believed it to be. The brain as the seat of consciousness is actually a fairly modern construct. As we've made that upward shift, we've also gone from being more spatial and embodied in our inner orientations to being very mental, linear, and abstract. We've shifted from feeling beings to thinking beings and supplanted intuitive thinking with rational-conceptual thinking. Overthinking is the extreme imbalance of this upward shift.

In terms of your overall energy supply, your brain uses around the equivalent of the defense budget of the United States just for its normal functions. If you're overthinking, your system will start taking the energy out of your body to fuel all that excess mental activity. The easiest way to know if you're overthinking is to look at the flow of your energy over the course of the day. If you hit the skids in the afternoon and need to fuel up on caffeine and sugar to stay alert, I can almost guarantee that your mind is running too many programs. You need to figure out what programs are using up the most battery power and start to close out those tabs.

These programs are overwhelmingly unproductive. Research has shown that people tend to think the same thoughts over and over again. We get really stuck in thought ruts, and then our mental energies continue to flow along those established pathways. A good visualization here is to imagine all these stupid, habitual, boring old thoughts that you think day in and day out written all over a chalkboard. Then I imagine myself taking a nice, big, fuzzy eraser to that chalkboard and wiping it clean. Try doing this every morning! Start the day with a clean slate. You can always write the thoughts back if you want.

To get control over your thinking mind, you have to first know that it's possible. Then, you need to know that the thinking mind is not as necessary as it would have you believe. Turning things around in your head over and over is not helping you to figure them out. Interrogate any beliefs that are driving overthinking. Do you believe that you have to "figure things out" to have your life work? Do you believe that you're supposed to be stressed all the time? Try the following mantras: *I acknowledge the subconscious belief that I need to be stressed. I am willing to release this belief. I open to the belief that I don't need to be stressed. I'm willing to trust life to unfold as it needs to without me worrying about it.*

When I was speaking about this with my son Cassidy, who is privy to all my wisdom, he told me, "Mom, I get it. But the voice in my head just keeps coming back." So how do we get rid of it? The reality is that this is not a problem with a quick-fix or speedy solution. It's taken me years to come into a place of authority over my own thoughts. There are certain aspects of the journey to healing and wholeness that require us to settle in for the long haul, and this is one of them. It's a commitment to your own sanity that creates change over time.

In the meantime, one of the best things that I have found to quiet the mind is the practice of deep listening, which can bring us into a calm, relaxed alpha brain wave state. I've had my brain waves recorded in an alpha brain wave state for minutes at a time, which is apparently fairly uncommon. I will be quite honest that the only reason I can go for minutes at a time without thinking is because I've spent years listening deeply to my tuning forks while working with others. My brain has been conditioned into an alpha state. Listening brings presence. Listen to the sounds around you. Listen to flowing water. Go outside and listen deeply to the sounds of nature. Listening brings us into concert with what is. Even listening to the sound of your neighbor's lawn mower is an opportunity to be in presence. You don't need headphones or an app or a teacher for that. Nature is in a state of ease and flow, and when we avail ourselves to that, we enter into that state. But you don't have to be in nature, either. Listening to music is also a great way to get out of a busy mind.

When it's difficult to settle the mind enough to just listen, another tactic is to consciously delete whatever program you're running and replace it with a more beneficial one. Override your own unbeneficial thought patterns! There are so many ways to use the mind constructively and creatively rather than destructively. We can use it to affirm how we're becoming healthier and freer. We can use it to love and praise ourselves. We can use it to pray. I don't consider myself religious, but I pray all the time. If I'm in the car and my mind starts wandering off, I'll turn my inner dialogue around and use it to pray for all beings everywhere to be free from suffering, or I send a prayer to wherever in the world it's most needed.

16

CROWN: Stepping into the Cosmic Dance

When our consciousness comes into balance all the way up at the crown, we really start to operate in a state of flow. We can hear the song of the universe ringing in our cells. At the crown center, we also move beyond our limited selves, beyond the ego and beyond the pain body, to experience our essential unity with all that is. We come into complete resonance with our own nature, which brings us into resonance with the collective field—the aether.

Sitting right on the top of the head, the crown chakra is our gateway to the unified field—the universal electromagnetic body. It draws in the positive flow of electrons through the Sun Star (that plasmoid sphere located around eight inches above your head). This is where we take in the energy of the sun and stars and all the cosmos. As that positive current of cosmic energy enters our inner battery terminal, it descends through the central channel, twirling around the ascending current of earth energy, exiting through the foot centers and circling around the outer boundary of the toroid back up to the crown. The crown is associated with the color white (or in some traditions, violet), the vowel sound "eeee," and, like the third eye, the seed syllable "OM" (or in some traditions, the silent pause after the sound of "om" is uttered).

When I first started doing this work, my understanding of the crown chakra was based on what I'd encountered in esoteric literature, which said that it was all about spirituality and our connection with the divine. In addition to this conventional wisdom, over the years, I've discovered that the crown also seems to hold energy related to our *relationship with time*. When I first observed this correlation, I didn't quite know what to make of it. Everything I'd read had told me that the crown was about God and higher consciousness. What the heck does time have to do with that? The connection started to become clear in my mind when I happened across the following quote: "Faith is knowing you have enough time to do everything you have to do." Here were faith and time in the same equation! Suddenly, I saw that we can only experience a sense of connection with nature and God and the universe if our minds are in a state of present-time awareness—meaning not only being fully present but flowing with divine timing, resonating with the movements of the aether. If we're rushing and distracted, worrying about the future, or fussing about the past, then we're not centered in the crown, and we're not in alignment with the flow of nature.

What does it feel like to be in right relationship with time? You flow through your day. You're not stressing about your to-do list. You don't get road rage. You're not anticipating what will come next. You're not at the mercy of your inner taskmaster. You find the appropriate balance of ease and effort. You're not swimming upstream. When you allow yourself to fall into your own right timing, there's a letting go that happens. You rest in the perfect geometry of nature. This is when you experience moments of magical synchronicity. You meet the right person at the right time. You get the perfect parking spot. You attract the opportunities you're seeking and the resources you need to make things happen. Someone buys you a pineapple. You play just the right tune in the greater symphony of life. It's actually a pretty blissful way to live!

Unlike the other energy centers, I do not find emotional information on either side of this center, but I definitely can find every age anyone ever had a head injury. The energy of the crown will also reveal if the person spends a lot of time under fluorescent lights, which can be highly damaging to the integrity of the double-layer plasma membrane at the top outer edge of the field—not to mention the sense of severance from the natural world that's created when we spend most of our days indoors under artificial lighting. In the glandular system, the crown is connected to the pituitary gland, the "master gland" located in the exact center of the brain, that produces a majority of the body's hormones and directs the entire glandular system, sending instructions that impact growth, digestion, sleep, blood pressure, and countless other physical functions. I have sometimes sensed into a cloudlike structure of false beliefs and illusions that surrounds the pituitary, that strikes me as a projection of falsehoods, clouding our perception and creating a felt sense of disconnection.

RELEASING PRESSURE VALVES

The chronic feeling that we don't have enough time is something that most of us live with, and it's a really tough burden to carry. When we're under time pressure, we are in constant struggle. It saps the joy and light-heartedness and creativity out of us faster than almost anything else.

Being *out* of alignment with time is something we often experience as an energy that pushes down on us, creating a feeling of being under pressure. When I've gone through periods of overwhelm in my life, the experience is a physical sense of pressure over my head. I've since observed this same kind of pressure in many other people's fields. It shows up in a contraction and condensing of the energy around the crown. In Biofield Tuning, the degree of resistance in the crown reflects the current level of pressure that the person is experiencing as well as the record of previous times in their life that they were under pressure. The force of contraction around the head is easily detected in the tone and vibration of the forks.

Being under pressure produces a layer of static on top of our healthy tonal expression. When a person's field is chronically under pressure, disease is the eventual result. Time pressure creates disease. Stress creates disease. It's when we are under time and money pressure or under the

244 | ELECTRIC BODY, ELECTRIC HEALTH

pressure of toxic relationships or a soul-sucking job or a huge tax bill that we blow *stress gaskets*. This is the term I use to describe what happens when you're under stress and a certain body part blows because that's your weak zone. We want to keep our bodies like a tight ship that has a full crew so that all tasks are completed and everything is humming and running at all times. Have you ever had to complete a huge work project when your team has three people out sick? That's what it feels like. Half the crew is absent. Over time, that kind of pressure can make your spleen or liver or another one of our stress gaskets give out.

You can also think of a state of pressure as too much electricity and not enough magnetism. Too much entropy and not enough syntropy. Too much gravity and not enough levity. Too much descending current and not enough ascending current. One simple thing you can do is take your shoes off and walk around with your feet on the grass to feel that levity rising up in you.

When we're struggling under the pressure of our own thought patterns and limiting beliefs, the antidote is to find the levity. For every downward force, there is a corresponding upward force. It's so important to find that uplift—you need a counterbalance to the difficult characters and situations that are weighing you down. Catch the updrafts! Throw off that time, money pressure, thought pressure! Most of the time, it's just the endless pressure created by the thinking mind. In many people, it shows up as what I call *storm clouds* around the head—turbulent thought forms blocking the flow of light and energy coming down through the crown. So much of mental and spiritual freedom is the release of this pressure, opening the valve, and letting the steam out.

Healing the crown requires us to rewrite our stories and beliefs of "not enough time." Over the years, I've heard a lot of: *Things are always so busy. I don't have time. There are too many things to do. I'm overwhelmed. I'm swamped. I can never catch up. If you're not busy, you're not being productive.* These are just stories that we need to interrogate and spin on their head. I invite you to deeply question your relationship to the story of "I don't have enough time." Is that how you're living your life, sometimes or all the time? How comfortable are you with the speed of your life? Do you believe that you have time to do all the things you need to do? Are you chronically rushing? Do you feel like you need to immediately respond to every text and email? What would it look like for you to live in a state of time abundance? Be willing to consider a different story about time: *I believe that I have enough time. I don't need to rush. I have time and energy enough for everything that needs to get done. I can accomplish more by doing less.*

"Not enough time" is just a state of mind. If you start to get into that state, you need to ask what can wait for tomorrow or the next day. If you're noticing that you're not in right relationship with time, take a look at your to-do list. What can wait? Do you really need to be putting this kind of pressure on yourself? Is it just a habit? There's a good chance that you are piling up all these things because feeling under pressure is just your habit. It's the comfort of your "known zone." But an honest appraisal of tasks usually reveals that something can wait. Catch the updraft rather than swimming against the current. Look at what you need to do, and choose to do the thing that feels best for you in the moment.

Contrary to popular belief, we do not become more effective, and we do not get more done when we get all amplified and accelerated. The old saying, "Haste makes waste" is very true, in my experience. Here again, we circle back to the root chakra's imbalance of guilt-driven overdoing, which leads to more doing and more stress—but not to more effective outcomes.

We want to have a clear and coherent relationship with time so that we're not getting all sped up and out in front of ourselves. One thing that I'm dogmatic about is never letting myself get all frothy and ahead of myself. I believe that this is truly one of the worst things we can do for our health. You can get a lot done without getting worked up about things. When something is feeling time crunchy, I just don't do it. That feeling of pressure and contraction tells me that it's not in alignment for me to try to squeeze it in.

I firmly believe that you can go the extra mile even while exerting the least effort. It's not about being half-assed in what you're doing, it's about being smart. I think you should do exactly what you need to do and nothing more. Otherwise, you're just wasting your energy. We want to soar and glide, not expend our energies carelessly by running around like a chicken with its head cut off. This also requires us to be centered not only in the crown but also the root, the center of right livelihood. It completes the circuit of our energy systems.

RIGHT RELATIONSHIP WITH TIME

Even if you've spent your whole life out of the now and in wrong relationship with time, it's not too late to come back to center. There are infinite ways to bring yourself back into the present moment. Figure out what works for you and make a practice around it. One of the most healing things for the crown chakra is to simply spend time in nature.

In Vermont, I've worked on a lot of hunters and loggers. They tend to have very smooth, healthy crown chakras because they're spending so much time in nature. They're out connecting with the elements, working with their hands, enjoying the peace of a quiet mind. They also tend to have a very healthy relationship with time. They're simply present in the moment and in their environment. They're not distracted or busy trying to get somewhere else.

We want to realign our inner compasses with the cycles of nature. Everything in nature has its own cycle. Nothing blooms all year round. There are times of birth, times of growth, times of decay, times of death, and times of rebirth. The stars are going around the galaxy, and the galaxy is going around the universe. It's all flowing in this perfect cosmic dance. Why do you need to rush? There's plenty of time!

Getting back into nature is the best way I know of to heal our relationship with time. Because ultimately, there is really no separating nature from time. The explicate universe is all about rhythms and cycles. The moon has a cycle around the earth, the earth has a cycle around the sun, and the sun has a cycle around the solar system. It's all just one big old space-time continuum. Flow is a state of connection with these larger cycles.

This is the wisdom of our ancestors that lives inside of us. The people who came before us knew instinctively how to live in harmony with nature. The ancients believed that every human being is a *microcosmos,* a reflection of the whole. You *are* the universe. It's all inside you. You are naturally aligned with the greater rhythm of life to the extent that you are operating from your true center, rather than some off-lying vibration of the pain body.

Modern humans have become disconnected from the rhythm of nature as we've synced our lives to artificial, accelerated rhythms. Our lives have sped up, and so have our bodies. Our heart rates have increased. Our brain waves have accelerated, too. Life on earth—including the human brain—has organized itself to the tune of the Schumann resonance, the organizing background rhythm of the ionosphere. That frequency, 7.83 Hz, is the frequency of our brain waves when we're on the alpha-beta brain wave cusp, in a state of presence, awareness, and quiet mind. It's a place that we get to in moments of meditation and deep stillness, and I believe that it's also our natural, default state of mind. But when we're riding the frequency of the thinking mind, which is in the high beta range of 13–16 Hz or more, we're in the accelerated electrical activity of the monkey mind that doesn't shut up. This is the very definition of stress. When you're under stress, your brain waves are accelerated, your nervous system shifts into fight or flight, your heart rate speeds up, and your blood pressure is higher. That's not a state of flow. That's not a state of blissful connection to nature and all that is.

When you're operating in flow with nature, you become a servant of the universe, guided and directed by a bigger plan beyond yourself. The secret to living the life of your dreams is not pushing and efforting to make all your dreams come true. It's about being free enough inside yourself that you can execute the dreams that the universe has for you. As you liberate yourself to follow your natural flow, anything becomes possible. As someone who has made a commitment to living life at the edge of creation, I'm telling you that the universe has far more amazing plans for you than you could ever concoct yourself—but those plans can only materialize if you can let go of forcing your own agenda.

This requires us to trust in life. Do you trust the flow of the stars, the sun, the moon, and the cycles of nature? Do you trust that you can step into that flow and allow it to guide you? In my experience, life knows what it's doing. Allowing myself to rest in my trust of the universe is like falling back into a big, comfy beanbag. I know that the universe has my back. Nature knows what's going on, and I don't have to try to figure it all out. What a relief! Even if things are happening that seem weird or difficult or wrong in the moment, I know that it is somehow for my good, even if I can't understand it right now.

ENTERING INTO THE COSMIC DANCE

With all our day-to-day stressors and problems and distractions, we blind ourselves to the wonders all around us. We forget how wacky, weird, and wonderful this whole scene is. What does it even mean to be human? What's going on with these bodies of ours? Instead of being in the wonder, delight, amazement, pleasure, joy, and playfulness of it all, we get all snarled up in our pain bodies. It's like being tangled in fishing line. You're so stuck in your own pain and your ancestors' pain, in your stories, your future and your past, that you're not able to stand in awe at the miracle of this human life.

A big part of the crown is really just a childlike wonder at the great mystery of being. You don't have to believe in God to open up your crown. It can also be about the perfect geometry of nature. When we attune ourselves through the crown chakra to the music of the spheres, to the deeper harmonies of creation, we can let this perfect geometrical flow of life inform our being. We can drink that in and let it nourish every cell in our bodies. I recently created a set of tuning forks based on the Fibonacci sequence. This sequence of numbers starts with 0 and 1, and each number is the sum of the two that came before it. If you divide a number by the one that came before it at any point in the sequence, you get roughly 1.618, or phi, also known as the *golden mean* or *golden ratio, which is also associated with beauty, truth, harmony, and the middle way.* Using these forks, which are 89 Hz and 144 Hz (the 11th and 12th positions in the sequence), informs us with the information of the perfect geometry that underlies the structure of our bodies and the world around us, and puts us in alignment with the essential harmonies of nature.

If you look at the earth and the stars and the galaxy, the whole celestial symphony—it's all perfect. Life is perfect. We've been programmed with all this noise that says that life is all a big, chaotic mess, and we're all guilty sinners fallen from grace. Meanwhile, stars are being born and flowers are blooming and the perfect dance of life is going on all around us. When did we start believing that we weren't a part of this dance? When did we start believing that life wasn't perfect? This is something for all of us to look at and reflect on. Where did that even come from, and why are we laboring under that illusion?

The illusion of separation is a deep imbalance that shows up around the crown chakra. This false perception of separation from the whole of life really blocks our flow. From an early age, we're taught to view the universe as machine rather than organism. We are separate from God, from nature, from the human family. That programming lives within us and informs us whether we know it or not. It's a very key, fundamental jam in our signal that shows up very prominently in the crown and the heart. And we had nothing to do with it! We were born into this story, and it's made us feel like we're alone in the universe. It generates what is called *Cartesian anxiety*: the deep-seated fear stemming from our belief in the fundamental separateness of everything.

In the field above the crown, I sometimes encounter a construct that is a kind of wall in the subconscious separating ourselves from the universe. Like any wall-type structure in our energy fields, it sucks huge amounts of juice out of us. See if this is something that's present in your own field, and if it is, try to envision it. Is it made up of concrete blocks? Is it steel? Stone? See how that wall appears to you in your mind's eye. Get curious about it, and then begin to explore what's on the other side. What kind of energy would come in if this wall weren't blocking it? Know that you have the ability to remove the wall. Then ask yourself: *What kind of action can I take in my own imagination to eliminate this? Do I smash it down? Do I roll over it with a bulldozer? Do I touch it and it just goes* poof *and it magically disappears?* Trust that whatever comes to you is a way of successfully knocking down any construct in your mind that's separating you from all that is.

Another image I've encountered while working on the crown is that of an inner antenna that picks up information from nature, God, the universe. The antenna is all wrapped up in a wad of duct tape that's blocking the signal. We can unwrap that duct tape and become a clear receiver again. All the garbage that's in the way—time pressure, beliefs in our own smallness and inadequacy, the illusion of separation—can be cleared out.

I tend to associate this cosmic antenna with the pituitary gland. The pituitary is highly sensitive to signal jammers around the head: cell phone towers, Wi-Fi, 60 Hz of electricity running through the walls. While that's certainly no reason to live in fear of technology or give your power away to things you can't control in your environment, it's just another reason to get your voltage up so that you can keep your signal strong and healthy no matter what. The signal of the pituitary gland also gets jammed up with illusions and false beliefs. This phenomenon took me by surprise during a group tuning session for autoimmunity. As I often do, I went into the session not knowing what part of the energy system I was going to work on, and I let the energy of the group tell me where I needed to go. At the start of this particular session, I got a note through my mail slot to work on the pituitary gland, which I'd never done a full session on before. What I found were these structures of illusion surrounding the pituitary gland, a cloud of false beliefs that was heavy, sludgy, and unbeneficial. It looked almost like a rotating panorama of different illusions. It felt like being stuck in the matrix and having your mind co-opted by a false view of reality.

You can develop a conscious practice of taking in the energy of the cosmos through your crown chakra and using it to fuel each of your energy centers as it descends the central channel. It's a visualization that I call the *rainbow body*.

Start by bringing your awareness into the crown, feeling a stream of white light flow down from the top of your head. Experience your central channel as a column of light. Open up to this feeling of the descending current mingling with the ascending current. As white light comes down through the crown, it splits through the prisms and into the different colors of the visible light spectrum. The diamond and all the gems that are in us. When we align with our rainbow bodies and geometry that informs that, it's like the static clearing from the radio, and beautiful music starts coming through so clearly. It's such a relief when the noise goes out of the signal. Come into that state of clear beingness. See the colors of each of your energy centers and know that you are a rainbow body of light. Feel into the inner illumination of your electric body. Remember that this light is the same light of all creation, of the whole universe. Through this light, through the central channel, you are connected to all that is.

HACKING BLISS

There's a programming that tells us that bliss and enlightenment (which are really one and the same) are unattainable. In my experience, they're not. As I've said, I don't think enlightenment is the elusive experience most of us have been programmed to think it is. I think it's just being aware of and resting comfortably in your light body. Enlightenment is experiencing yourself from the inside out as a being of pure light that is connected to all other beings. You are a marriage of heaven and earth! You're mud and minerals, and you're also starlight. You are the aether. When you awaken to that awareness of your own essential illuminated nature, you start to see yourself that way more and more. And when you connect to your own electromagnetic body, you connect to the universal electromagnetic body as well. You resonate with your own true nature and then you come into resonance with capital-N Nature. You start vibing with the whole. That's bliss! This experience is available to us, not at some point in the future when we're more spiritually advanced and eating a raw vegan diet but right here and now.

We get scared to surrender to these immersive, overwhelming good feelings because we're afraid that something is going to come along and push us back down to reality (as in, the familiar reality of our pain bodies). We won't even let ourselves go there because we're so afraid that it will be taken away. And this is true—it will be taken away. Life happens.

But you can enjoy it while it's there, and you can always go back and drum it up some more. But we can stay, for longer and longer periods of time with practice, in a coherent heart space. It is possible to spend most of our days and even lives in a state of love and gratitude for ourselves and others and all of life. That is a sustainable and energy-efficient state that we can achieve and live from. It took me years of clearing out the trash within myself, but I did it. We all can.

When I first came to understand space as one big electromagnetic organism and to know that everything that powers the stars powers my own heart and brain, I had a visceral experience of the song of the universe ringing in my cells. I felt on the deepest possible level that I was connected to the entire universe. For me, the awareness of my own light body connected to all things in one big field of light was what did it. I didn't need to search anymore. For you, it might be something completely different that gets you there. But all roads lead to Rome. What we're looking for is that visceral feeling of at-oneness with all of creation. That is true liberation of our spirit and ecstatic union with that which is greater than ourselves.

This, I believe, is the ultimate that we can experience as human beings. It's lofty and humble at the same time. From a biofield perspective, it's simply what happens when all the noise and junk are gone and you are free to vibrate at your own unique frequency signature. That's enlightenment, liberation, awakening, or whatever else you want to call it.

We are all diamonds on the inside. We're faceted and shimmering and reflecting all kinds of light in every direction. That crystalline experience of self—living in the pure radiance of our own light bodies, unburdened by all the heavy inputs we've been dealing with—is our birthright. We have to go on a bit of an archeological dig to get there, because that light has been buried for generations. We have to dig through the crap of generations of illusion and disempowerment and incoherent waveforms. But the gold that we uncover is an experience of our authentic selves. When you can rest in your true self, you become an instrument of the universe—a clear note in the symphony of creation.

You have the ability to enter into a state of unity consciousness with all of creation. You can connect with the aether, the unified field of infinite possibilities, through the vehicle of your own aetheric body. I leave this with you as a reference point so that you know that it's possible, not at some point on the horizon but right here and now.

LAST WORD: We Are the Ones We've Been Waiting For

We are experiencing a turning of the ages in which the old patterns are breaking down and a new pattern is being birthed. Everywhere in our culture, the old stories are unraveling and new ones are being written. This can be a scary and chaotic process, and many of us feel deeply the suffering that is occurring at this moment in history. But as the study of cymatics shows, when the frequency changes, the old pattern falls apart and a new and completely different pattern spontaneously emerges. Even if all we can see is apparent chaos and destruction, when we attune ourselves to the new frequency, we start to see the new pattern that is arising.

In our individual lives, it is much the same. When our frequency changes, there is a period of chaos as our old, familiar patterning gives way to a new and more aligned expression. Chaos precedes a new order. This is healing, growth, and evolution. Gradually, we let go of the noise of the pain body and tune ourselves more and more to our own fundamental frequency.

Everyone has in themselves the programming to rise to the occasion of what seems to be an emergency situation on Spaceship Earth. In this new paradigm, we have the tools to solve our problems individually but also collectively. What if everyone was tapped into their own greatness and didn't feel unworthy of stepping into the role that they were meant to play at this time? What if everyone was empowered to shine their light to make a difference? The solutions to all our problems are inside us—we just need to activate our ability to engage those solutions.

The resources are at hand! They're here, right now. In shamanic cultures, they believe that every disease has a cure in nature. God doesn't create any illness without also creating the cure. It's the same with our problems; for every problem, there is a solution. But we will only see the solutions if we believe that they're there.

Nature contains the codes that we are looking for. It's all there waiting for us to attune ourselves to it. The information for us to heal ourselves and our planet, to solve our individual and collective problems, is around us all the time if we're open to it. When we open our eyes to the electrical nature of our bodies and all of life, we open up to receive a multitude of new solutions. There is light, connectivity, and energy all around us to be tapped into and harnessed at any moment. The infinite potential of the unified field, the intelligence of Nature, is available to us should we choose to ask—and choose to receive.

And remember: Right here, right now is as cool as it's ever going to be! Stop moping around. If it's the end of the world (and I'm not saying it is), then let's enjoy ourselves with the time we have left! If the environment is collapsing and there's very little we can do about it, then let's at least enjoy ourselves, our bodies, each other, and our planet. And maybe, just maybe, by taking that turn of surrendering into pleasure and presence, we can turn things around. But we're not going to turn things around by sitting and moping about it and being in despair.

Life is meant to be celebrated. Nature shows us how to do that. Nature is abundant, harmonious, loving, and joyful. Living in a natural state of joy (bliss, even) is a revolutionary act. We have to be rebels of bliss, warriors of love, speakers of truth. That is how we counter the darkness in our world today—and what an incredible mission that is! The fight of our lives is the fight to bring beauty, harmony, and truth back to our lives and back to the earth. It doesn't have to be a struggle. It can be a great adventure. It's the deeper purpose and calling we've all been searching for. All you have to do is consciously raise your voltage and show up, radiating your light out through your own field and far beyond.

When you do that, who knows what miracles the universe is waiting to create through you?

APPENDIX A

FIFTEEN SIMPLE WAYS TO RAISE YOUR VOLTAGE

Get enough rest. This is the most important thing. Say *no* to running around when what you really need to do is rest. Avoid whenever possible pushing yourself through things, or making yourself go out for a run when you are exhausted. As a Chinese proverb says, "Want to live a long life? Take naps." Ideally, sleep from 10:00 p.m. to 6:00 a.m.

Breathe more deeply. Our primary source of energy is the breath. Start to notice when you are holding your breath, and make a point to take a series of long strong breaths. Make the *aaaahhh* sound on the exhale. Ideally we take full, easy belly breaths all day long.

Get grounded. While there are many products out there like grounding sheets and mats, nothing beats bare feet on the ground. If you are in a cold climate or can't get outside, wear socks or non-rubber-soled shoes while you're inside.

Eat whole, pure, fresh foods as often as you can. It is the embodied sunlight, the electromagnetic energy we get from food, that nourishes our electric bodies. Refined, packaged food contains little to no life force or nutrients.

Drink spring water, or ideally, structured water or charged water. There are many devices out there for making water that is superior to the dead, chemical-laden water that unfortunately comes from most taps.

Consciously *receive* **love and gratitude and appreciation.** These energies that others are seeking to give you are a currency. Don't say *no* to them. You are worthy.

Hang out with electron donors, not electron stealers, whenever possible. Seek to become an electron donor yourself by making sure you are doing your best to meet your own needs.

Allow your emotions to flow through you rather than suppressing them. Give yourself space to find healthy ways to express these waves, remembering they will pass.

Tap into the power of sound. Make use of listening to energizing music, singing, chanting, toning, and dancing.

Get out in nature. Go for walks, forest bathe, listen to birds, get near moving water, and breathe in ionized air.

Laugh. Laughter is the best medicine. Watch or read funny things, hang out with funny friends, practice cracking yourself up.

Honor your natural inclinations. Give yourself permission to do what feels right and natural to you in the moment.

Choose "ahh" over "uggh." Choose doing things that make you feel uplifted over things that make you feel downtrodden whenever possible.

Avoid chemically scented candles, detergents, and other products. Chemical scents are being called the "new tobacco" and have been implicated in many health issues.

Soak up the sun. Get out in the sun, without sunscreen on, every day. Adequate sunlight is vitally important to maintain proper voltage levels in our systems.

APPENDIX B

BIOFIELD TUNING
biofieldtuning.com

Biofield Anatomy
Significance of Energetic Imbalances

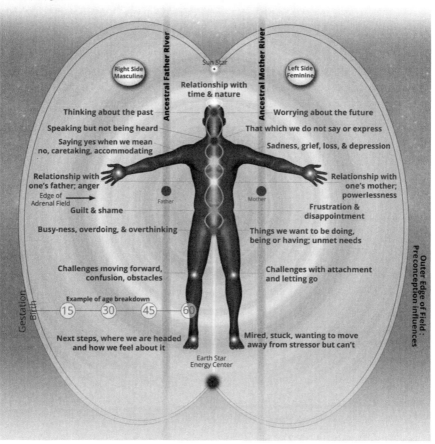

APPENDIX C

RESOURCES

Biofield Tuning: Learn about classes, tools, practitioners, and virtual sessions on our websites.

- www.biofieldtuning.com
- www.biofieldtuningstore.com
- www.sonicslider.com
- www.electricheath.com

Researchers and Experts

Dr. Zach Bush, triple-board-certified physician, microbiome expert, and regenerative agriculture advocate (https://zachbushmd.com/)

Dr Rashid A Buttar, surgeon, author of *The 9 Steps to Keep the Doctor Away* and Medical Director for the Centers for Advanced Medicine (https://www.AdvancedMedicine.com and https://www.CentersFor AdvancedMedicine.com)

Reverend Tiffany Barsotti, Biofield Science and Energy Healing, www .healandthrive.com

Dr. Jack Kruse, neurosurgeon, health educator, and founder of Kruse Longevity Center (https://jackkruse.com/)

Dr. Dietrich Klinghardt, founder of the Klinghardt Academy, the American Academy of Neural Therapy, medical director of the Institute of Neurobiology, and lead clinician at the Sophia Health Institute (http://www.klinghardtacademy.com/BioData/Dr-Dietrich-Klinghardt-MD-PhD.html)

Dr. Claude Swanson, MIT-educated physicist and author of *Life Force: The Scientific Basis*

Dr. Gerald Pollack, University of Washington bioengineer, author of *The Fourth Phase of Water* and *Cells, Gels, and the Engines of Life* (https://www.pollacklab.org)

Dr. James Oschman, biophysicist, author of *Energy Medicine: The Scientific Basis* and *Energy Medicine in Therapeutics and Human Performance*

Dr. Jerry Tennant, ophthalmologist, author of *Healing Is Voltage* and other books (https://www.tennantinstitute.com/)

Dr. Beverly Rubik, biophysicist, founder of the Institute for Frontier Science (https://www.brubik.com/)

Dr. Bruce Lipton, stem cell biologist, author of *The Biology of Belief* and other books (https://www.brucelipton.com/)

Dr. Rupert Sheldrake, biologist and author of *The Science Delusion, Morphic Resonance,* and other books (https://www.sheldrake.org/)

Dr. Sue Morter, bioenergetics researcher, founder of the Morter Institute, author of *The Energy Codes* (https://drsuemorter.com/)

Dr. Glenn Streeter, exercise physiologist and energy medicine practitioner (https://www.energymedfit.com/)

Jonathan Goldman, sound therapist, author of *The Humming Effect* and other books (https://www.healingsounds.com/)

John Beaulieu, sound healer and researcher, author of *Human Tuning* and other books (https://www.johnbeaulieu.com/)

Books

Tuning the Human Biofield: Healing with Vibrational Sound Therapy by Eileen Day McKusick

The Invisible Rainbow: A History of Electricity and Life by Arthur Firstenberg

The Body Electric: Electromagnetism and the Foundation of Life by Robert O. Becker

The Electric Sky by Donald Scott

Electric Nutrition: A Revolutionary Approach to Eating That Awakens the Body's Electrical Energy by Denie and Shelley Hiestand

The Lightness of Being: Mass, Ether, and the Unification of Forces by Frank Wilczek

Life Force: The Scientific Basis by Claude Swanson

Anatomy of the Spirit by Carolyn Myss

My Stroke of Insight by Jill Bolte Taylor

The Fourth Phase of Water by Gerald Pollack

Healing is Voltage by Jerry Tennant

Energy Medicine: The Scientific Basis by James Oschman

The Biology of Belief by Bruce Lipton

The Subtle Body by Cyndi Dale

Energy Medicine by Donna Eden

Vibrational Medicine by Richard Gerber

Becoming Supernatural by Joe Dispenza

Real Magic by Dean Radin

The Energy Codes by Sue Morter

Energy Medicine Yoga by Lauren Walker

Online Events and Summits

The Body Electric Summit: https://bodyelectricsummit.com/

Reuniting Science and Spirituality Summit: https://reunitingscienceandspirituality.com/

Ancestral Healing Summit: https://ancestralhealingsummit.com/

Sound Healing Global Summit: https://soundhealingglobalsummit.com/

INDEX

horse, 188
Human Design system, 88
human reproduction, 40
Hunt, Valerie, 66
hyperactivity, 139–40
hypotheses, 30–31
  Biofield Anatomy Hypothesis, 17–18,
    30–31
  biophoton, 71–74

illness, chronic, xxii
illumination, 56–58
imbalances
  adrenal, 187
  biofield anatomy, *263*
  third eye, 228
immune system, 109, 110, 118, 137, 178
inclinations, natural, 260
indecision, 117
inner coach, 159
inner critic, 157–59, 237
inner sun, 170–71
instantaneous communication, 52, 67
Institute of Noetic Sciences (IONS), 30–31
intention, 99, 102, 170, 171, 217, 226
  awareness and, 29, 99, 104–6
  power of, 107, 185
  science of, 53, 66
  stuckness and, 124
  visualizations on, 182
intergenerational trauma, 29–30
intuition, 76, 81, 227, 230–31
IONS. *See* Institute of Noetic Sciences

Jain, Shamini, 67
Jamaica, 224–25
jazz music, 218
journey, xxxiv–xxxv
  authors, 4–8
  healing, 108, 239

kettle corn, 12, 15
Kidney 1 point (K1), 113
Klinghardt, Dietrich, 72

knees
  in biofield anatomy, 122–25
  as holographic, 124
  left, 129–32
  right, 126–29
"known zone," leaving, 114–17

laughter, 260
leaving "known zone," 114–17
left foot, 117–21
left knee, 129–32
left side
  of heart chakra, 199–201
  of root chakra, 143–45
  of sacral chakra, 159–61
  of solar plexus, 174–77
  of third eye, 235–37
  of throat chakra, 214–17
levity, 34, 244
L-fields, 65
light, xv, 43, 55–56, 72–74
  awareness of, xiv, 42
  body, 59, 252
  fluorescent, 242–43
The Lightness of Being (Wilczek), 47
Lipton, Bruce, 76–77
listening, 218–19, 220, 239
livelihood, right, 145–46
liver, 168, 172, 173
localized patterns, 25
loud spots, tuning forks detecting, 12–13
love, 192–94, 201, 206–7, 260
low voltage, xxii

magnetic fields, 20, 80–81
"magnetic fluid," 64
magnetic sense, 229–33
magnetoreception, 231–32
magnetosphere, 36, 37, 81
manifestation, 224–25
mantras, 107, 239
map, biofield, *19, 28*
Marley, Bob, 97
Martin, Howard, 60
mastiff, 142

ABOUT THE AUTHOR

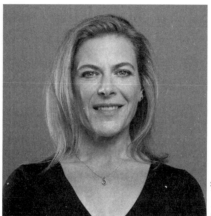

Erica Allen

Eileen Day McKusick is a pioneering researcher in the fields of electric health and therapeutic sound. She is the creator of the sound therapy method Biofield Tuning, founder of the Biofield Tuning Institute and Tuners Without Borders, and author of the bestselling, award-winning book *Tuning the Human Biofield: Healing with Vibrational Sound Therapy.*